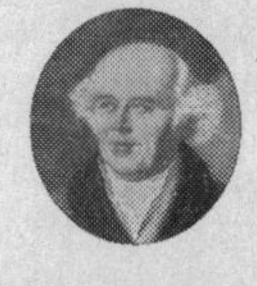

WELCOME HOMEOPATHY

Dr. S. C. Madan
M.B.B.S., F.R,C.S. (U.K.) M.N.C.H. (U.S.A.)
SENIOR E.N.T. CONSULTANT
HEAD OF E.N.T. TROMSO (NORWAY)
FORMERLY SENIOR E.N.T., CONSULTANT (U.K.)

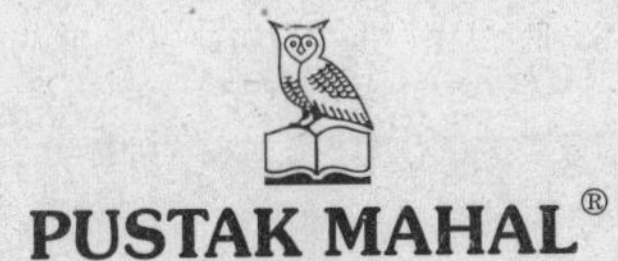

PUSTAK MAHAL®

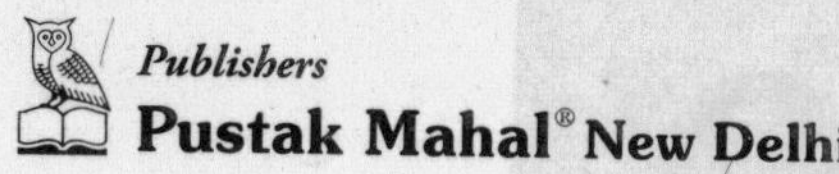

Administrative office and sale centre

J-3/16 , Daryaganj, New Delhi-110002
☎ 23276539, 23272783, 23272784 • *Fax:* 011-23260518
E-mail: info@pustakmahal.com • *Website:* www.pustakmahal.com

Branches
Bengaluru: ☎ 080-22234025 • *Telefax:* 080-22240209
E-mail: pustakmahalblr@gmail.com
Mumbai: ☎ 022-22010941, 022-22053387
E-mail: unicornbooksmumbai@gmail.com
Patna: ☎ 0612-3294193 • *Telefax:* 0612-2302719
E-mail: rapidexptn@gmail.com

ISBN 978-81-223-1137-2

Edition: 2016

Printed at : AR Emm International, Delhi

Preface

Dear Readers,

At the outset, let me thank all of you for the wonderful support you have lent me every time. I am overwhelmed at the response I got from all of you, not only from remote corners of India, but also from countries like U.S.A., Middle East and Canada. Needless to say, if it had not been for all of your repeated requests and pleas to dwell into more types of illnesses cured by homeopathy, I would probably have not yet got the impetus to proceed with the making of this new book "Welcome Homeopathy".

I am repeatedly faced with the queries as to my choice of homeopathy, in spite of being an allopath (ENT surgeon) by profession. My reply is echoed in the following article in which Dr E. Henry Smalpage– a renowned surgeon has written about his 'conversion' to this field of medicine. Coincidently, I happened to read this and it would be injustice on my part not to share it with all of you:

'............................Maybe, I am the only Fellow of the Royal College of Surgeons of England, who, after the most intensive training in surgery, has deserted not only surgery but also all forms of allopathy, to enter the realm of homeopathy. And clearly, after the experiences of such practice, with no small reputation for surgical skill, I must have had very strong reasons for casting all these aside to enter, like a new student, into a field in which I was then a complete ignoramus but also, like most allopaths, one who openly condemned homeopathy as absurd and even worse.

If any man ever had to eat his own condemning words, I did. But the results have been in many instances very satisfying, if not for the pocket and allopathic friendships, at least for the mind and spirit.

As everyone can realise, it needed what seemed to me to be a miracle to convert a highly successful surgeon – if success can be measured in money and public applause – into a renegade – a homeopath.

A boy of eleven years of age was brought by ambulance from his home many miles away from my city consulting rooms. He had been in and out of many allopathic hospitals, under the care of many allopathic physicians, famed and not so famed, for over seven years, for a condition of the spinal nerve centres, which brought about often repeated convulsions of the body and lower limbs. Nothing all the allopaths could do had ever produced any beneficial results, so the possibility that I could do any better by similar methods was remote. As the ambulance men lifted the child from the stretcher to place him upon my examination couch, he went into a condition of clonic spasms with his back drawn into a state of opisthotonos – that is, drawn back until the back of his head was closely approximate to the back of his legs – a condition which is characteristic of acute strychnine poisoning. But this condition had recurred many hundreds of times over the preceding seven years.

Obviously as an allopath, I had no possible remedy. But Homeopathy did have the remedy – Tinc. Nucis Vomicae – homeopathically potentised, and I happened by chance to have the 30th potency of this drug. Its use was dramatic. Within a few minutes, the terrible spasms, which I was told usually went on for as long as thirty minutes, completely disappeared, but miraculously still, with repetition of the same therapy three times daily for one month, there were no spasms, and the boy – now twenty years older – has made and retained a complete recovery.

Then, as the Directing Fates ordained, a few days after seeing this first seeming homeopathic miracle – where allopathy for several long years had proved its complete futility – I had a very well known citizen of Sydney with an excruciating painful right orchitis due to violent contact of that part of his anatomy with the sharp edge of his open motorcar door. I have never had such an experience personally, and never want what the man went through, until homeopathic Pulsatilla 6x - one dose daily – after two futile morphine injections by an Allopath – completely changed the whole painful picture by completely removing all the pain and within one hour, the man, previously confined to his bed in agony, left for his business office in the city with the simple instructions to repeat the Pulsatilla every three hours, which he did for the rest of that day – three doses only – and that was all. Two days later, he rang me up to say that his condition had almost returned back to normal.

That was good. But I was still a sceptical allopath. Then a veritable lifesaving miracle almost completely shattered any of my remaining doubts. A man, 65 years of age, was brought to my consulting rooms – as I had ceased to visit patients' homes – with a high temperature, a running toxic pulse, and an obviously highly inflamed appendix, but also with a cardiac condition which made surgical intervention seemingly deadly. I gave that man, more through desperation than faith, the homeopathic Belladona 6. I repeated it three times at quarter hour intervals. Then, being pressed by other patients who were waiting, I sent him home with instructions to repeat the Belladona therapy and ring me during the late afternoon. I received two telephone calls – one to say the patient was greatly improved – the other by his local doctor to abuse me for losing him a surgical operation and its fee.

The next case I consider a veritable life saving miracle. And I can say without any fear of reasonable contradiction that a fine young man now twenty years of age and soon to graduate as an allopathic doctor, the only one to enter medical profession in Australia, would never have passed through his first few days of his life without homeopathy and the so-called coincidence that I was in the maternity hospital where he was born and in which death for him seemed then inevitable and only a matter of hours.

Two hours after he was born – without drug or artificial mechanical meddling – he had a rectal temperature of 106 degrees, and was burning hot with an intense dry heat, and for two hours all the efforts of his skilled allopathic obstetric surgeon and nursing sister to save him had proved futile.

The dry burning heat, the fast approaching mortality and the fact that the little victim sipped a little water only, from a spoon, then turned its head slowly away and then back to sip again, left no doubt in my mind that if homeopathy was to win a victory over impending death, potentised Arsenicum Alb. was the indicated lifesaver. Arsenicum Alb. 6x – a few drops well diluted in water – was given in a few drops, every few minutes. In fifteen minutes from the first dose, the rectal temperature was normal, and the otherwise doomed child made a complete recovery – strangely enough – saved from death by homeopathy when allopathy had proved futile – to spend six years of his later life filling his mind with futile allopathy so that when graduated as a medical man he could cast aside and forget what he had been taught by his allopathic teachers to embrace the Art of Homeopathy to which alone he owed his salvation from near death.

These were my introduction to Homeopathy – enough, most people will agree, to drive me into seeking to know more of this allopathically condemned « Nonsense » or « Quackery ».

Twenty years have now passed, and with them my extensive consulting surgical practice has died its just death.

The four emergency cases presented prove the marvel of homeopathic cures.............’

Coming back to this book, this 4th edition is on the same pattern as the 3rd edition of this book but it differs a lot from the 3rd edition in that it deals with completely different diseases from those mentioned in the previous edition.

This new edition deals with more complicated cases where allopathic treatment has failed and side-effects of allopathic treatment are worse than the disease for which allopathic treatment had been given.

I have dealt with common diseases which are in epidemic proportions as follows:

Thyroid, polycystic ovaries, menstrual irregularities, autoimmune diseases like rheumatoid arthritis, ulcerative colitis, thyroid diseases, multiple sclerosis

The intractable diseases like multiple sclerosis where allopathy has hardly anything to offer.

Tumours like lipoma, fibroplipoma where allopathy is almost always a failure, have been successfully treated with homeopathy.

Cosmetic ailments like, small breasts, pendulous breasts, facial hair in women has been treated– provided not already spoilt by hormones and laser treatment. Pigmentation of facial skin, chloasma has been treated – as given under Plastic Surgery (Cosmetic Homeopathy)

Recurrent urinary infection in women, vulvovaginitis responded beautifully to homeopathy.

I have not failed to mention the successful antidotes to the side-effects caused by the necessary post-angioplasty/post cardiac surgery medications as well as also the anti-tubercular medicines.

Arthritis –where methotrexate and steroids and NSAID preparations have played havoc.

Emotional diseases like teenagers' depression, anxiety, anger, hyper-irritability, obsessive compulsive disorders (OCD), religious insanity in women especially at menopause-leading to separation and divorce.

Gym exercises and computer related illnesses have been dealt with.

Gastritis and gastric reflux where H.pylori kit has caused side-effects.

Spinal diseases like low backache with partial paralysis of lower limbs, Cervical spondylosis have been treated with homeopathy.

Deafness and meniere's (vertigo, noises and deafness) where all allopathics across the globe have failed, homeopathy with expertise have given excellent results.

Nasobronchial allergy and Bronchial Asthma, pollen and dust allergy and also eye diseases like chalazion, retinal diseases, post cataract ailments have been dealt with.

Finally, I would like to make some acknowledgements from my side.

I am highly indebted to Dr Sridharan, Medical Director, Holy Family Hospital, Delhi– a renowned cardiologist and physician, who constantly encouraged me during writing this book– for he bears no prejudice to other branches of Pathy (Homeo, Allo, Natural) as long as the treatment is safe and with good results.

I am extremely obliged to Dr. Kulbhushan Bharadwaj– equally distinguished homeopathic physician who, apart from his speciality of Homeopathy having extensive knowledge of other branches like Naturopathy and Ayurvedic, has spared his precious time to give healthy criticism in this book.

Challenging cases brought by Dr Ashok Sharma of Mathura, having in-depth knowledge of all the branches of medicine (Homeo, Ayurvedic and Unani) have widened my experiences in dealing with complicated cases.

I am much obliged to my nephews –Vicky Tendon and Manish Grover who taught me the art of simplifying the computer writing of my book.

I am extremely grateful to Dr. Leena Mendiratta-microbiologist of Apollo Hospital, Delhi, for making the necessary corrections of my book.

I can never forget my obligation to Mr. A. P. Gulati, Under-Secretary Govt. of India (retd.) who initiates me and acts as a guide to me, in homeopathy.

I sincerely express a deep sense of gratitude to the publishers of the book for their cooperation and hard work.

S. C. Madan

Ph.: 9958372312

Foreword I

It gives me great pleasure to write a foreword for this book by Dr. S. C. Madan.

Just as in foods they say, 'One man's meat is another man's poison', in Medicine too what seems to work for one person does not necessarily work for the other.

Unfortunately in allopathy while we recognise this different responses by patients, our treatment regimes are more disease orientated rather than person orientated. Homeopathy is one science that pays a lot of attention to the individual patient and treatments are fine-tuned to his/her needs and therefore while diseases may be the same,the treatments may not always be the same.

Dr. Madan has utilised his allopathic training to fine-tune his mind to make the right diagnosis and then decide which system of medicine he thinks would work best for a patient and then offer the same. With the passing years, his experience seems to reflect that homeopathy has a lot to offer and with measure of success he has achieved, he feels that if practised well this could offer succour to many more people.

It is with this intention Dr. Madan has written this book and the hope is that people will take more responsibility over their own health, pay attention to initial symptoms which could be relieved by the medicines that the book is suggesting and thus prevent major catastrophes in the future. However, do keep in mind that these are guidelines and general rules and one should never hesitate to get in touch with Dr. Madan, if the response is not as expected or wherever there are any doubts.

Dr. Madan's selflessness and his dedication are to be admired and I am sure that his efforts to dissipate his knowledge and experience will go a long way in helping patients who always need the right guidance.

I wish him well and wish the book great success.

Dr. S. K. Sridharan MD
Medical Superintendent
Holy Family Hospital
New Delhi 110025

Foreword II

It gives me immense pleasure to write the foreword second time to Dr. S.C. Madan's second book - WELCOME HOMEOPATHY. The first book 'Homeopathy Cures Where Allopathy Fails' has been a thumping success. Dr. Madan has received appreciation for the same from far and wide, personally and telephonically. Many people have been since consulting him for their problems of the soul and finding great relief. The main reason for that, he being an Allopath basically, has been applying his knowledge of Allopathy making him little distinct from others. I have seen Dr. Subhash Madan using Homoeopathic remedies pre and post surgery as an adjunct therapy because he believes that the use of Allopathic medicines which have their side effects are minimised and is able to achieve good results.

According to the principle of homeopathy, every case needs individualisation, and therefore the services of the physician cannot be ruled out. However, with regular practice and experience in contact with majority of the cases, the near specifics are always categorised. What makes Dr Madan's approach different is his experience based on his earlier success of unique combinations and diagnosis of patients based on etiopathology– the core of allopathy.

In this volume, many chapters have been added by him which would be of interest to the lay-professional and lovers of Homeopathic science. Much hard work has been done on them and the application of Homeopathy has given Dr. Madan complete success in these new areas. This book

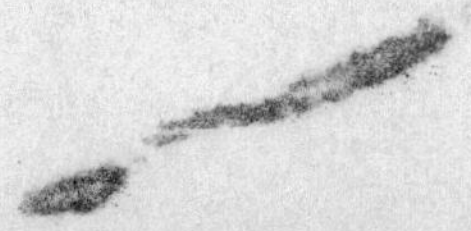

has special chapters on Mental diseases, Plastic medicine, Dentistry, Ophthalmology, Thyroid, and Polycystic ovaries.

Dr. Subhash Madan and myself share a close professional relationship so we share our clinical experiences with each other and on that basis I can say that the remedies and treatments mentioned in this book for various diseases are almost time-tested. I wish this book a great success and interesting reading for all the lovers of Homeopathy.

Dr. Kulbhushan Bharadwaj
M.H.C., D.H.M.S.; Dc.G.M.; M.L.H.I.(Geneva)
C - 23841212

Index to Welcome Homeopathy

1.

SKIN DISEASES

ACNE

This is one of the most daunting skin ailment affecting mostly young adolescents and early middle-aged women. The females get superadded emotional depression because of being more conscious of their cosmetic appearance than men.

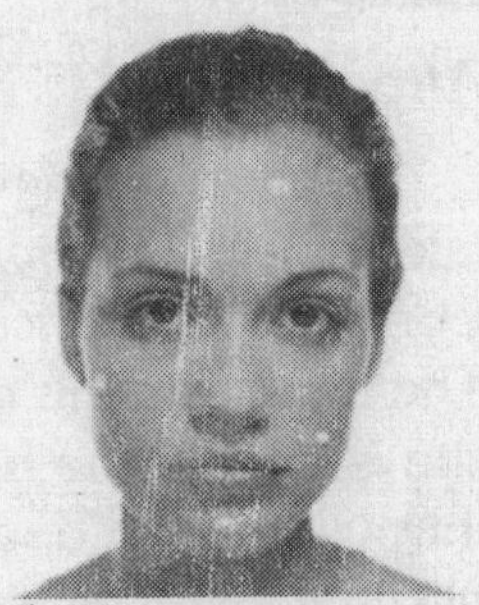
Lady with **acne** on her face.

With modern rich oily food and fizzy drinks, this condition is becoming more common.

Also most of the young girls are put on hormonal treatment for irregular periods and these hormonal preparations are notorious for causing acne.

I was flabbergasted to see some of the very rich patients, after spending thousands of dollars on imported medicine for use and have landed into serious life-threatening side effects.

Case-1

Allopathy:

This young business lady came to me for Hirsutism (facial hair), depression, both of these symptoms she developed after the use of co-cyprindiol.

She was also complaining of leg cramps since she started this medication. On my examination, she had developed Thrombophlebitis also because of this remedy.

The depressing thing was that acne was still persistent as before.

Homeopathy & A.C.T:

I treated her depression with Aurum met & Ignatia.

I treated her acne with Ant.crud. and Pulsatilla

I treated her Thrombophlebitis with Belladonna and Hammemelis.

Case-2

Allopathy:

Another young woman who had acne had imported the latest medicine by the name of Roaccutane (Isotretinoin). Considering its price, she thought it will do magic to her acne. The mother of this girl came along with her, told me that since she is taking, she has become very irritable and has become introverted and does not mix up with her friends. I diagnosed her that she is getting depression as one of the side effect of Roaccutane.

On my further questioning, the mother told me that she tried to commit suicide since she has been on this medication. This girl was also getting bald– again the side-effect of Roaccutane.

The above two cases demonstrate the side-effects of so-called 'Scientifically' proved drugs by these protagonists of Allopathy.

Homeopathy & A.C.T:

This case has come to me recently. First I am treating her depression before I go to her acne and irregular periods.

SKIN ALLERGY (Severe Eczema)

Recently I had two severe cases of chronic eczema and Lichen planus of hands and feet.

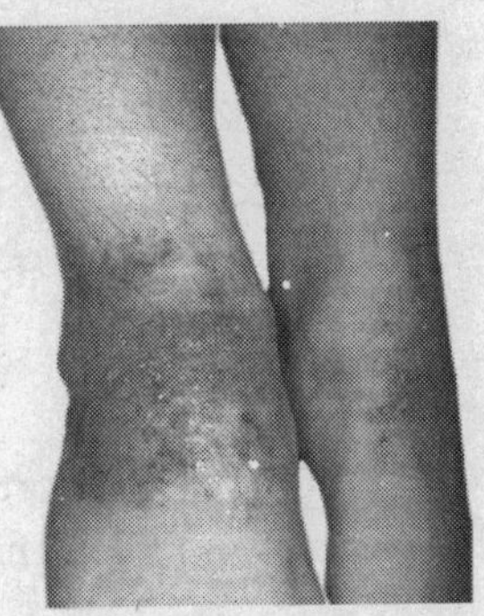

Skin allergy on legs.

Case-1

He was treated by topmost dermatologists both at Apollo and AIIMS, Delhi. The treatment after taking repeated biopsies which showed no malignancy, but simply chronic inflammation.

Allopathy:

The treatment for three years revolved around the same, i.e., steroid, antifungal and antibacterial creams along with antibiotics orally from time to time. If the condition became worst due to allergy to antibiotics, then he was put on antihistamine and steroids which lead to further dryness of skin. By the time he came to me, the skin of hands and feet was like parchment and cracking.

Homeopathy:

1. I asked the patient to stop Dettol soap immediately and completely

2. I gave calendula and Hypericum cream to apply

3. Advised him to avoid nylon socks as these with sweating were making proper culture media for fungus and bacteria.

Internally, I gave him:

Alumina 200 in morning (due to dryness of skin) Kali arsenicum 200 noon and Staph.200 at night (due to his violent temperament)

It took me 4 months to cure this patient.

Case-2

He was another apparently very similar to case no. 1 in every aspect, but in this case I could elicit different cause for his chronic eczema.

He had chronic sinus infection, but he was more bothered about his skin than occasional headache or letharginess due to sinus infection.

Allopathy:

I operated upon his sinuses and thick viscid pus was drained, then I put him on:

Homeopathy:

Hydratsis and acid Fluor. And Calendula and Hypericum cream to be applied locally.

He was cured in four months.

A.C.T.(Author's Comments & Treatment):

I will request my allopathic colleagues to go into the cause of any ailment rather than generalising allergy and giving antiallergic treatment leading to more complications, whether it is skin, chest or nose allergy.

Equally, I will request Homeo colleagues to be careful in prescribing Sulphur in high potencies in allergic cases. I have seen patients coming with severe aggravation getting allergic to the name of Homeopathy.

CRUSTA LACTEA
(Seborrhoea of scalp in children)

This is a very common condition in infants and newly born children.

Allopathic treatment of this condition plays havoc with the child for years as evidenced in the following case. Many such cases have come to me.

Case-1

18-month-old son of doctor parents came to me with severe eczema of scalp. They had already visited the reputed dermatologists who had advised steroid cream and when the allergy shifted to chest by this suppression, then the child was given systemic steroids.

Case-2

Like the above case, bronchial asthma in this child was so severe after applying steroid lotions that he was given systemic steroids for two years by the Director of Immunology and was always suffering from eczema and bronchial asthma and he got hair on the face and typical cushing's syndrome.

Homeopathy:

On the basis of the fact that child developed crusta lacteal after BCG vaccination.

I started treatment with thuja and calarea carb (lot of head sweating) followed by Mezerium and natrum sulph (getting worse during rainy season).

All external applications were stopped. Budecort nebulisers had to be continued for sometime before finally stopping these altogether.

FRECKLES (Lentigo)

These are small pigmented or whitish lines or patches on the cheeks. These often occur due to either exposure to sunrays or due to hormonal changes after pregnancy.

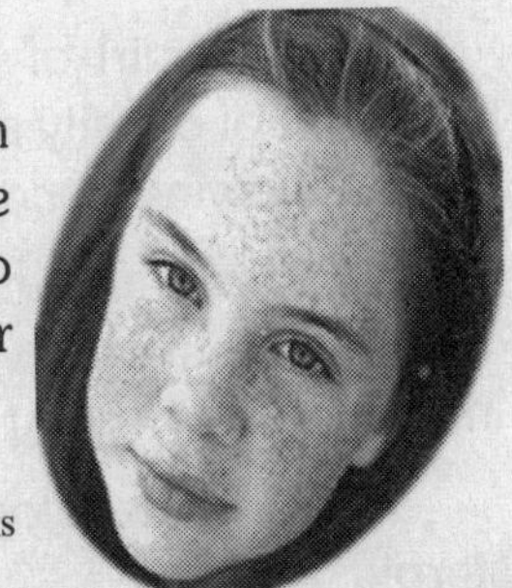

Whitish lines or patches on the cheeks

Allopathy:

I find the results after laser are sometimes very discouraging due to overshooting the intended results.

Regarding treatment at beauty parlours, that is anybody's guess as to how far the results will be permanent.

Homeopathy:

Sepia especially in women is of unquestionable value.

If there are warts also, then acid nitric especially in middle-aged dark complexion women have never let me down.

URTICARIA

It is a challenging and frightening condition owing to the fact that it may go into Anaphylactic Shock, which is life-threatening.

In this book, I will mention two interesting and challenging cases and these are eye openers to allopaths as to how its treatment with allopathic medicines lead to lot of complications, which are often irreversible.

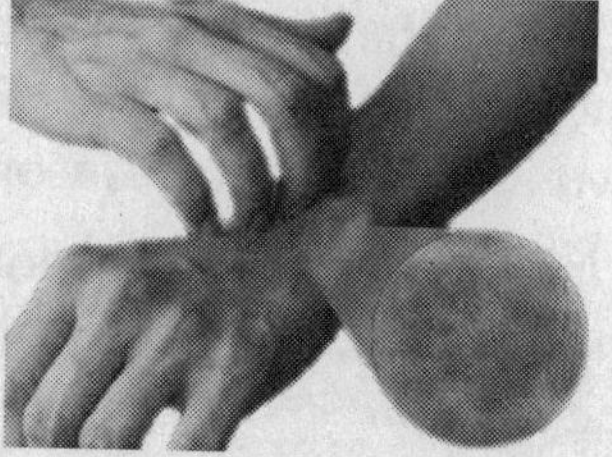

Urticaria

Case-1

A young girl of 28 years, from Bangalore came for her treatment of obesity and irregular periods after taking treatment of the following in consecutive order:

A few months after the delivery of her child, she started developing urticaria for which she was given steroids by injection followed by mouth steroids.

Then she developed irregular periods and obesity due to steroids.

For the treatment of irregular periods, she was given hormonal preparation by one after the other obstetricians, basically the same hormones.

Whenever she wanted to stop hormones knowing the side-effects (being an educated lady) she would not get periods.

Then she developed depression due to obesity and secondary amenorrhoea.

She was given antidepressant treatment, which further lead to increase in weight.

That is the stage she came to me after she happened to read my last edition of the book.

Homeopathy:

I started the treatment first, by giving Thuja 1000, since she developed rash during pregnancy because of being given tetanus vaccine, which no doubt is a routine procedure as a safeguard.

Then I uplifted her depression: by Ignatia and Aurum met.

Thereafter, I treated her cushing's syndrome which was due to steroids by natrum sulph and apis.

Then I treated for her irregular periods with sepia, pulsatilla and cimcifuga.

Now after six-month-treatment, she is cheerful, with regular periods and a slim beauty, looking half the age than what she looked when she came to me.

HAIR FALL (alopecia)

This condition of patchy hair fall or partial or complete baldness is becoming very common owing to the following causes:

1. Strong hair shampoos do not prevent hair fall, rather causes hair fall due to strong chemicals.

2. Vaccinations these days have become the cause of premature grey hair or hair fall.
3. Stress and anxiety is another common cause of hair fall.
4. Dandruff is another cause. The dandruff itself is due to modern fashion of keeping the hair dry or using too many hair conditioners.
5. Severe illness or strong antibiotics is another cause of hair fall.
6. In my observation, hypothyroid– which itself is due to ovarian dysfunction, is caused by giving hormones by the gynae obstetricians at the slightest stroke of irregularity of periods.

Allopathy:

Various local preparations can hardly be of any permanent benefit.

Hair transplant apart from the cost does not give a natural look.

Homeopathy:

According to the aetiology, I have dealt such cases by the following remedies:

1. Vaccinations side-effect have been dealt with thuja.
2. Mild homeopathic dandruff shampoo with kali sulph internally has given very good results.
3. Stress and strain have been dealt with kali phos and ignitia.

It is a common observation these days that unlike 30 years ago, hair fall and premature greying of hair is becoming extremely common.

Many factors are responsible for its side effect of fall and greyishness of hair.

1. The common cause which many dermatalogists do not realise, numerous vaccinations which are responsible for its side effect of fall and greyishness of hair.
2. The other common cause is strong shampoos which because of its strong chemical ingredient for dandruff cause hair fall, since many patients have given the history that it has happened soon after applying shampoo.
3. Dyeing of hair even with so-called natural mehendi, for colouring, since even that contains strong chemicals.
4. Certain hair conditioners and certain chemicals used to straighten or curl the hair are responsible for hair fall and premature greying of hair.

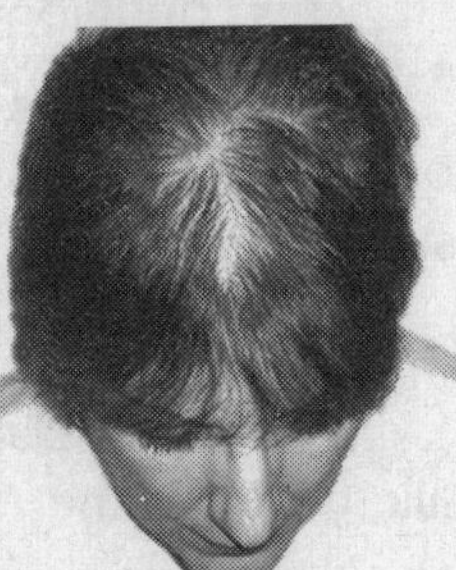
Hair fall

The following case histories have confirmend my view point:

Case-1

Allopathy:

A young boy was brought to me with complete alopecia. The boy had patchy alopecia at age of 3-4 years when he consulted the topmost dermatologist at a reputed hospital of Delhi.

This dermatologist made the case worse to its maximum, by giving growth hormones which increased the growth physically but made the alopecia complete.

The worst still after spending lot of money of the patient on repeated hormones caused steroid side effects.

Homeopathy:

It has taken me six months before he started growing his hair under homeopathic treatment which was as follows. At the time of print, the patient is still under my treatment.

The Lesson: Be wary of strong shampoos and colouring and dying agents, and also the agents used for curling or uncurling of hair.

BEDSORES

This condition is a bugbear to the medical profession.

Recently I was asked to treat a challenging case of bedsores of 70-year-old female who developed bedsores after spinal surgery and became incontinent for stools and urine.

She was allergic to most antibiotics.

Even local Betadine could not be applied since she was allergic to iodine.

Homeopathy:

I cured her bedsores with calendula and hypericum ointment rather than calendula powder, since her skin was extremely dry due to cetrizine given for allergic reactions.

Her urine incontinence I treated with argentum nitrate and lac. The results were excellent.

ITCHING

This is one of the most annoying nonfatal condition.

Allopathy:

The common treatment irrespective of the site or underlying condition is giving anti-allergic (levocetrizine), if the worst ten steroids is the line of treatment.

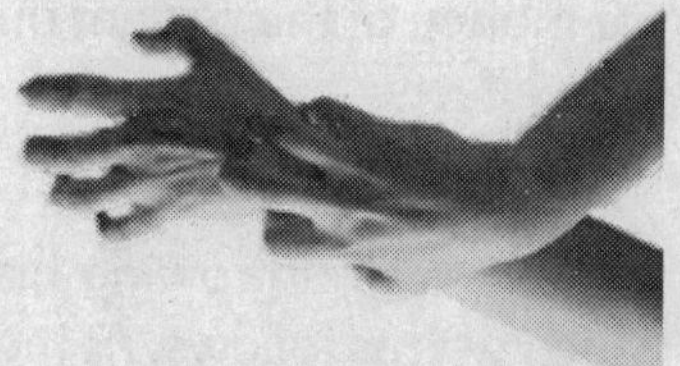

Itching

I have seen patients who are treated this way leads to suppression of underlying condition which is not easy to unmask then.

To make matters worse, local creams containing steroids, antifungal, anti-allergic, anti-inflammatory is nothing but a smokescreen against fire. The moment you stop using this steroid cream, the itching or eczema comes back again.

Homeopathy:

In infants and children, atopic dermatitis due to vaccinations is dealt with thuja and mezerium. Other conditions of itching is dealt with arsenic alb and apis.

Conditions arising in cold weather and if associated with rheumatism are dealt with rhus with excellent results.

Vulvovaginitis itching is dealt with ambra and sepia.

The worst cases of itching are dealt with graphites, but only in experienced hands.

Itching due to allergic reaction with certain foods are best dealt with apis, arsenic and antimonium crudum

Severe itching with extremely bad temper, tendency to swear, staphysagaria gives excellent results.

◆◆◆

2.

DENTAL DISEASES AND DISEASES CAUSED BY DENTISTS (UNINTENTIONALLY)

DENTISTRY 1

There is very little I have mentioned about dental ailments in my first book. But since the publication of my first book, I have seen hoards of ear, nose and throat ailments caused by dental surgeons, neither by negligence nor intentionally.

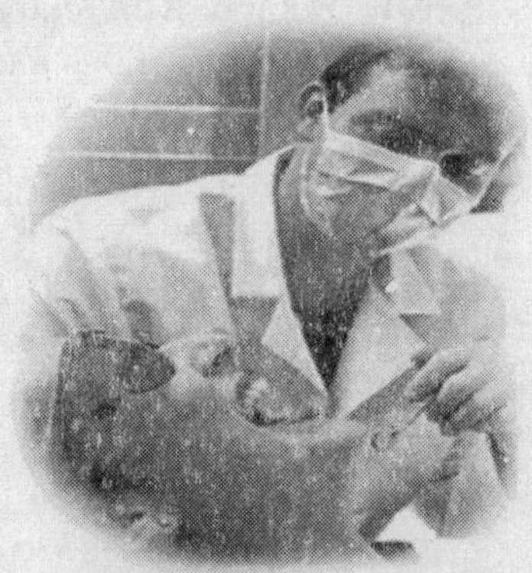

Dentist examining the patient

The following chapter will certainly invite criticism from my professional dental colleagues, but there is no prejudice against them or their professional capabilities, as I have used the word unintentionally. All the cases mentioned give lessons from which we can take precautions.

Case-1

This is a typical case amongst the hundreds that I have seen. A young lady of 45 years, after root canal treatment was having mouth ulcers and lymphadenitis of the neck.

She had no ulcers before the dental treatment.

Allopathy:

The dental surgeon had given loads of vit.C for the ulcers and Brufen for the pain.

The local application was Zytee which is aspirin in gel form. She was also given antibiotics - Erythromycin.

No relief, so she was sent to me.

Homeopathy:

I gave her merc sol, borax and belladonna alternating in cyclic rotation.

She showed improvement in three days.

A.C.T(Author's comments and treatment):

These ulcers are caused by dentists because they inject local anaesthetic (Xylocaine with Adrenaline) before dental treatment. If the quantity injected is more (depending upon the need of the patient), then there is vasoconstriction of blood vessels leading to denuding the blood supply of delicate mucous membrane.

To make matters worse, they give Brufen which is notorious for causing mouth ulcers. So sometimes without any infection, there is associated cervical lymphadenitis due to aseptic inflammation of mucous membrane of mouth.

I came to this practical conclusion when there used to be ulceration of nasal mucous membrane after smr operations, if we inject more of this vasoconstrictor; hence, even in nasal operations I use more of normal saline than too much of adrenaline.

DENTISTRY 2

Dentistry & Temperomandibular Joint:

A. I have endless list of patients directly or referred by dentists because of pain in front of the ear, around the ear, at times going towards the temple region of the head.

At other times, pain in or around the ear while chewing food.

Many times wisdom tooth has been extracted in such patients with these symptoms.

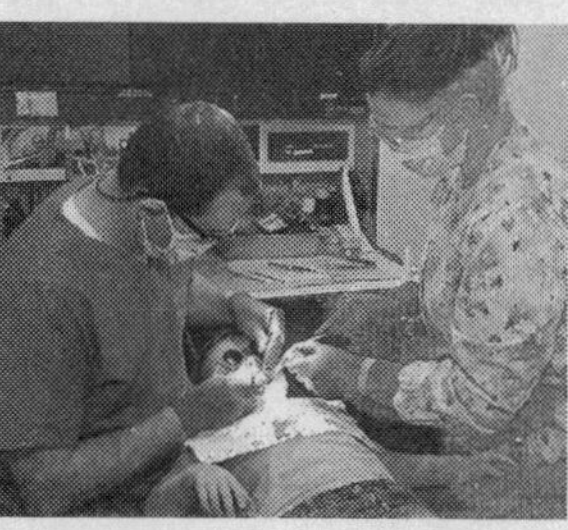

Dentist examining the patient

In all the patients with the above symptoms, I have mentioned the underlying disease was due to dysfunction of T.M. (temperomandibular joint)—the joint in front of the ear.

In ninety per cent of such cases, the dysfunction is caused by dentists (due apologies) not by negligence, not intentionally, without realising that they have been caused by dental treatment.

Again, majority of dentists miss this diagnosis as the cause of pain in that region (mentioned in above cases).

B. The other types of cases on the increase are patients who cannot close the mouth properly and the lower jaw falls during sleep. This is due to subluxation (loosening) of T.M. joint.

A.C.T (Author's comments and treatment):

Aetiology:

As to how the above two anomalies are caused is explained in the following lines.

In A category, there occurs fibrosis and loss of elasticity of ligaments of T.M. joint because of some dental treatment done earlier, months or years ago.

The onset is gradual and insidious and patients do not correlate with dental treatment and often have forgotten about it. The mechanism of the development of this pathology is that the mouth has been kept open far too long or opened very widely to allow the dental treatment, as a result the ligaments and cartilage of this joint are overstretched. It also depends upon the pre-existing elasticity of ligaments. Patients having generalised arthritis are more prone than with normal joints.

The other important point to be noted is patients come with the complaint in the opposite joint and not the side of the joint having had the treatment done. This is explained by the fact that patients chew the food on the opposite of treatment for a few days or weeks, owing to pain and swelling on the side of treatment. This leads to imbalance and joints dysfunction.

This just like standing on one knee, while the other knee had the injury.This leads to osteoarthritis of normal joint.

Diagnosis:

In all the above, categories can be confirmed by plain X-ray and CT scan.

Allopathy:

Often they give Brufen or other anti-inflammatory drugs which cause mouth ulcers, which lead to cervical adenitis—the stage at which most patients have come to me.

Homeopathy:

A Category of patients, I give cal. Fluor and Causticum.

B Category of patients, I give Arg. Metallicum and Ruta (cartilage and ligament involved).

In addition to homeopathic treatment, therapeutic ultrasound (in physiotherapy dept.) to the joint works likes a magic.

DENTISTRY 3

Case-1:

52-year-old lady came through one of my treated patient, with symptoms of pain in front of her left ear, radiating towards the temple.

She had dental treatment by best dental surgeons of Delhi and Mumbai where she originally comes from.

Allopathy:

After taking painkillers, first for root canal treatment, then for pain around left T.M. joint, she got the following 'gifts' of allopathic treatment:

1. She had severe gastritis despite taking antacids.
2. She developed piles for which she had Colonoscopy done.
3. She developed mouth ulcers and thrush in the mouth as a result of antibiotics and NSAID preparations. For thrush, she was given local steroid preparations and Metronidazole by mouth. She developed severe stomatitis because of Metrondizole.

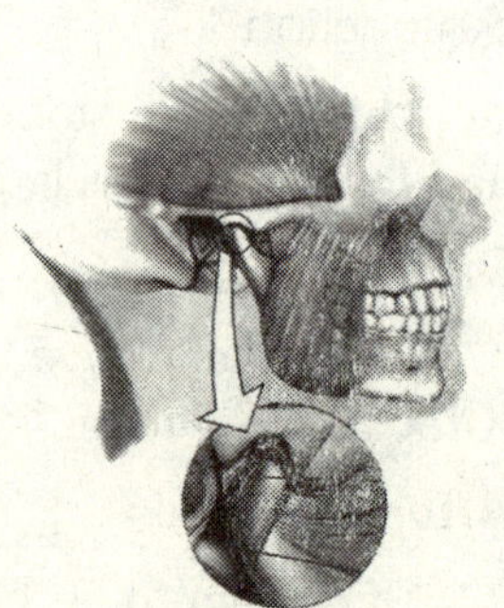

T. M. Joint

Homeopathy:

For T.M. Joint Dysfunction, I gave Ruta, Oxalic acid and Spigelia.

Reason for giving these homeo preparations was the ligament involvement and secondly the pain was on left side.

For Mouth Ulcers: merc sol and Borax

For Gastritis: Natrum phos + carbo veg

For Piles: Nitric acid and hamemmelis

DENTISTRY 4

Trigeminal neuralgia versus dental pain versus sinus:

This is an interesting case of a young man who had sinus pain in the region of left upper cheek.

He had the root canal done for the pain but no relief; then had the tooth extracted to relieve the pain but the pain still persisted. Then he was given strong painkillers for two years before he came to me feeling miserable with pain and side effect of painkillers.

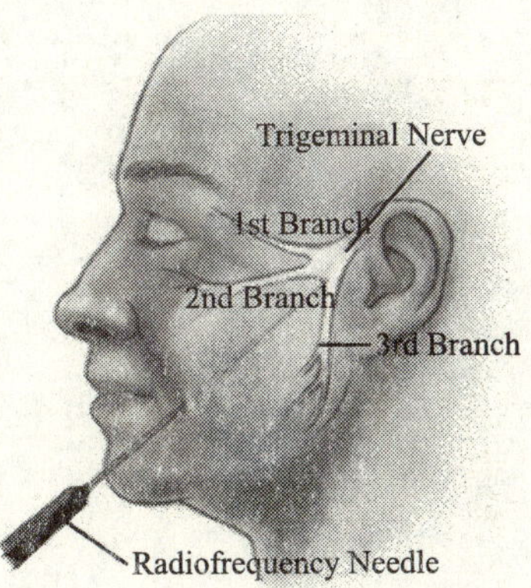

I had the X-ray of sinuses which showed opacity of left sinus and clinically severe trigeminal neuralgia due to dental treatment.

Homeopathy:

I gave him for left trigeminal neuralgia and left sinus treatment as below:

A. Spigelia+bell+mezerium+plantago major and chamomilla

B. Kalibio+acid Fluor+bell

The patient had dramatic improvement in two days which he had not had in two years with:

Allopathic:

Treatment after going to neurologist with: tegratol, diclogesic which played havoc with his stomach.

My advice to the dentists is to always exclude sinus infection– especially the teeth related sinus (premolar and 1st molar).

◆◆◆

3.

RESPIRATORY DISEASES

I will be dealing with only the allergic part of nose and chest allergy and not the infection part.

Although in the last edition I had mentioned in details about asthma and allergic rhinitis, but I am compelled to write in case the readers of this book who do not get the last edition miss this important subject.

ALLERGIC RHINITIS

Every third person these days attribute their sneezing and running nose to allergy.

Even the ENT surgeons find it convenient diagnosis and simple treatment to write antihistaminics, if patients do not respond, then steroid inhaler or nasal spray. However, I have found 90% have underlying sinus infection by the time they consult the ENT surgeon.

Advising Antihistaminics–levo cetrizine, alerid, allegra or any of their sister medicine, simply prolong the treatment and are only a smokescreen against fire, without treating the cause.

These simply cause stagnation and cause the sinus, nasal and bronchial secretions viscid, leading to sinusitis and bronchial asthma.

Steroid treatment, unless in status asthmaticus, in my experience mask the symptoms and do not treat the cause, and make these patients permanent customer of the doctor.

The other important point I wish to bring home to paediatricians, chest specialists, immunologists and ENT surgeons, that very often the aetiology in children asthma is vaccinations and decongestants (triominics, decongestants like these various cough syrups).

In adults, the common cause of bronchial asthma is chronic sinus infection, although the patient forgets these symptoms by the time he goes to the specialist.

The common treatment advised by ENT surgeons for sinusitis is cetrzine or allegra or other decongestants. These preparations worsen the sinus in the long run and cause bronchial asthma for reasons mentioned earlier.

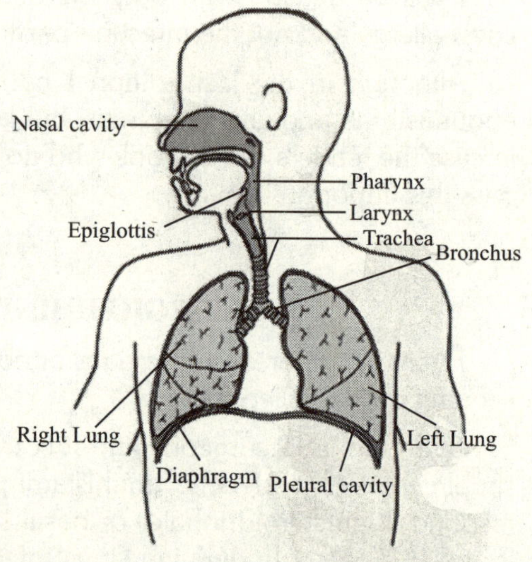

Homeopathy:

ACT(Author's comments and treatment):

Infants and Children Asthma: Without countering the side effects of vaccinations and without anti-doting the side-effects of anti-allergic allopathic and steroid drugs, you cannot cure bronchial asthma, or sinus infection or glu (middle ear effusion).

The infection part I treat with antibiotics, but the allergic part I treat with homeopathy.

In advance and chronic cases, I surgically remove infection from sinuses followed by drainage.

Medicine (allopathic or homeopathic) depending on the stage of disease.

It is essential to note that women developing asthma at menopause need completely different treatment depending upon their nature (irritability), sexual desires and religious rituals dealing with *dhoopbati*, *agarbati* etc.

In very elderly people with cardiac and bronchial asthma, I find arsenic iodide and ammonium bromide are of exceptional value.

Emotional asthma is not to be dealt with allopathic tranquillisers such as alprax and alzolam which in the long-term are habit forming and cause depression, but give them homeopathic preparations like anacardium and agnatia.

◆◆◆

4.

EAR, NOSE AND THROAT

MOUTH ULCERS (STOMATITIS)

This is a very common condition at any age.

One should try to find the cause rather than treating on symptoms.

Allopathy:

Gelora or zytee are not worth mentioning in my experience. These may give symptomatic relief but will not treat the cause.

Following are often the causes of mouth ulcers.

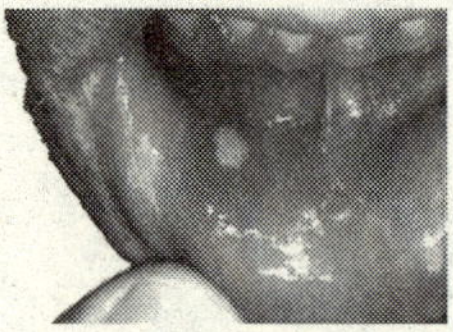

1. In infants and children,teething with diarrhoea are the common cause.
2. Bad orodental hygiene with gingivitis is another common cause.
3. Trauma due to artificial denture.

Mouth Ulcers

4. Gastrointestinal disturbances.
5. Strong painkillers or antibiotics.
6. Sinus infection is another common cause.
7. Another important cause of stomatitis which goes unnoticed and dental surgeons do not realise that they are responsible for this type of stomatitis.

a. By injecting vasoconstrictor like adrenaline with xylocaine. This denudes the blood supply of oral mucosa when the quantity is injected too much or patient's resistance is poor or patient is diabetic.

b. Second favourite of dental surgeons is metronisazole for gingivitis and for anaerobes, which cause stomatitis.

c. Painkillers like brufen, combiflam, flexon are the common medicines prescribed by dentists which cause mouth ulcers.

My treatment in such cases is folic acid by injections along with lactobacil and heavy doses of vit.C.

Homeopathy:

Merc sol, borax and kali mur are of unquestionable value.

These must be supplemented with probiotic (lactobacil especially acidophilus) and folic acid which is very helpful.

In very resistant cases, I have seen only nitric acid has worked.

In respiratory diseases, I would like to emphasise the point that lot of children have sinus infections with enlarged adenoids or adenitis, which lead to mouth breathing and eventually to dental (orthodontic) problems. It is a pity that in India even 1% of paediatricians do not lay importance to sinus infection as the cause of snoring, mouth breathing and repeated bad throats.

In U.K., I operated six such children with sinus infection and they had a magic relief in their respiratory and throat and ear symptoms. The irony of the fact is that even ENT surgeons in India do not attach any importance to sinus infection in children below the age of five years.

The usual treatment of these children with cold and cough is done by giving antihistaminic in one or the other forms (Cetrizine, Levoctrizine, Alerid, Alerid-D).

These preparations are simply a smokescreen against fire and do not treat the cause, and on the other hand cause stagnation and potential cases of sinusitis.

GLU EARS
(Middle Ear Effusion)

This is a very common condition among school going children, owing to frequent colds, bad throat and swimming.

Their eustachian canal is short wide and horizontal, so the infection travels quickly compared to adults.

The Antihistaminics given for cold and cough is another common cause of glu ears, by causing stagnation of secretions due to its drying effect. Many paediatricians and ENT surgeons do not realise this is the causative factor also. Rather they give antiallergics for every cold whether it is allergic in nature or not.

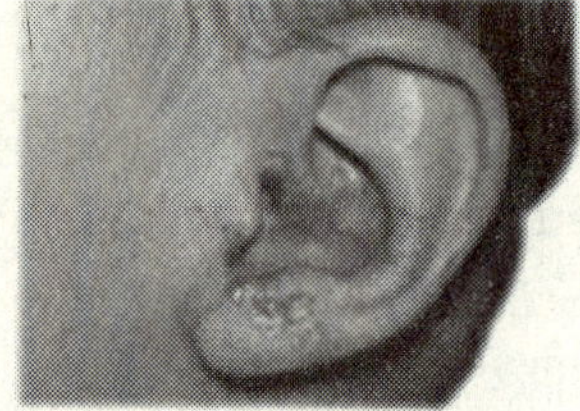

Middle Ear Effusion

The other pitiable thing is the ailment goes unnoticed by paediatricians who examine the ear as an eye-wash.

In India, I find it is the school teachers who complain to parents that their child is not attentive, only then it is brought to notice of ENT surgeons.

Tympanometry confirms the diagnosis apart from examination of ear by ENT surgeon.

Allopathy:

Operation followed by mucolytic agents, otherwise it will recur again.

It is paradoxical that in India most ENT surgeons will give cetrizen or allegra even after operation, which will cause recurrence rather than cure.

Homeopathy:

Merc. dulcis and kali mur is of unquestionable value.

CHRONIC MIDDLE EAR DISEASE
(Chronic otitis media)

This disease is a challenge to ENT surgeons even after radical surgery. Recently I had treated two cases who have been getting discharge from the ear after two mastoid operations.

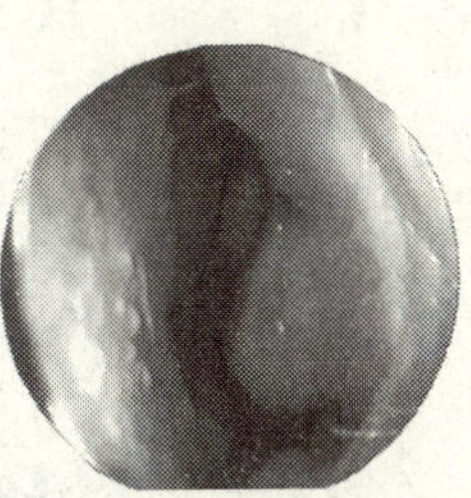

Chronic middle ear disease

Case-1:

In this case a girl of 12 years from Gorakhpur was having blood stained ear discharge, so I gave Lapis alb and acid nitric. Her ear was absolutely dry for six months after having two months treatment.

Case-2:

In this case of chronic Mastoiditis, there was foul smell of bone destructions. So I gave acid fluor and his ear dried up in 4 weeks time.

Inner Ear: Many cases of Meniere's disease, and Tinnitus are increasing day by day owing to extensive use of aspirin and anti-arthritic drugs.

Homeopathy:

I have treated vertigo with Carboneum sulphate and Chenopodium.

Severe cases of vertigo I have treated with Cocculus since in most of these cases there is element of fear, hence Cocculus has given very good results.

Other highly stung people I have treated with Theridion and phosphorus.

Cases of bachelors or married with sexual frustration having vertigo, I have treated with conium.

HOARSENESS OF VOICE

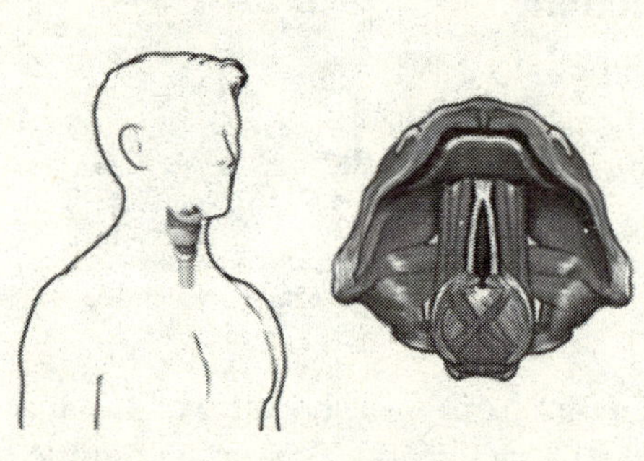

Throat Infection

Although I have dealt with this subject in the previous book, but since the previous publication, I have come across more resistant cases, after having allopathic treatment from reputed ENT surgeons in Mumbai and from voice hospital in Maharashtra.

I would like to stress the point that treating such conditions merely on symptoms does not give satisfactory results.

After examination of larynx and relevant investigations assisted by symptoms I gave the following treatment.

Case-1:

A missionary sister came to me after having treatment at various hospitals in Bihar and Kolkata with extremely hoarse voice and no relief.

Allopathy:

Every ENT surgeon was giving her anti-allergic (alerid, cetrizine, vozet alerid-D) after doing the videoscopy of larynx, thus impressing the patient that everything is fine.

I fail to understand as to why the patients do not ask the doctor that if the investigations are normal why the hoarseness is persistent.

In my experience as ENT surgeon, all antiallergics and decongestants increase hoarseness by making the normal respiratory secretions more viscid. This missionary sister was being given these medicines whether it was Mumbai or Bihar.

Homeopathy:

I gave one dose of causticum 1M and asked to stop all decongestants and anti-allergics and advised her to follow with carbo-veg 200 2-3 times a day and to see me in 5 days time.

To my surprise she phoned the next day saying that 'puree' has worked like a magic.

Case-2:

A school teacher having hoarseness of voice, after seeing three ENT surgeons in Delhi was told she has got vocal nodules and has to be operated upon but there was no guarantee that these will not recur. Moreover, there are chances that voice could become rougher after operation.

It reminded me of a case of litigation against three ENT surgeons in U.K. where the singer (the patient) sued that her voice had become rougher after the operation, however she lost the case as the surgeons did not promise that voice will become normal.

I treated this case on the basis of strain to the ligament of vocal cord, by giving ruta and arnica, and the patient made complete recovery.

Conclusion:

Always take aetio-pathology and relevant investigations into consideration, apart from symptoms.

Case-3:

Every resistant type of hoarseness in a teacher came to her after having seen the topmost ENT surgeons in Delhi at reputed hospitals who gave her the following treatments.

Allopathy:

Professor and Director of ENT treated her with antiallergic (cetrizen) and antacids (pantoprazole) basing his treatment on the basis of acidity and allergy which was causing the hoarseness.

May I remind my ENT colleagues that due to the drying effect of antihiataminics and also cf antacids, the hoarseness was not getting better.

Due to the profession of a teacher, there was strain on vocal cords and she at times used to experience pain while speaking.

To make matters worse, the director of ENT gave anti-inflammatory-brufen which was nothing but a smokescreen against fire.

Repeated endoscopies did not make any difference.

She was seen by two homeopaths, without any result, who probably treated on symptoms alone.

Homeopathy (A.C.T.):

I gave homeopathy on the basis of aetiology:

1. Arnica and ruta because of strain on vocal cord ligament-as a teacher.

2. Carboveg on basis of acidity causing hoarseness due to reflux. She was fond of chillies.

3. Phosphorus owing to allergic nature of her nose and larynx for which she was taking antiallergics for years leading to present state.

It took me four weeks to cure her.

Case-4:

This is an interesting case and most resistant type of hoarseness.

It demonstrates my viewpoint that treatment should not be symptom based only as most homeopaths do.

It also demonstrates that due to the side effects of allopathic medicines, though based on aetiology, these allopaths cannot effect the cure.

The lady of 40 years, teacher by profession came with severe hoarseness of 4 years duration, with no improvement after seeing three top ENT surgeons in Delhi and four reputed homeopaths in Mumbai and Delhi.

Allopathy:

ENT surgeons gave her antiallergics (cetrizine, alerid, allegra) and at times painkillers like brufen if she had pain while straining her voice. She was also being given antacids to counteract acidity, as she had lot of acid reflux also which no doubt can contribute to hoarseness.

The diagnosis by all the ENT surgeons was the same, chronic laryngitis with tendency to nodule formation.

I would like to ask three questions from those reputed ENT surgeons:

1. Do not they know that antiallergics cause dryness of salivary secretions and increase viscosity of saliva, thus leading to more hoarseness.

2. Antacids like pantoprazole and omenaprazole also cause dryness of saliva thus further leading to hoarseness.

3. Strangely the patient had no allergic element in her larynx.

4. No ENT surgeons among three of them had gone into details of her acidity.

Coming to the four homeopaths who had given remedies on the basis of symptoms alone were as follows:

Causticum, arg.met, cal.fl, nux vomica.

Homeopathy (Author's Comments and Treatment): I gave homeopathy based on examination of larynx and history and symptoms:

1. The patient used to take lot of red and green chillies which was causing acid reflux. I asked her to stop that and gave her carbo veg.

2. I excluded sinus infection by exam and X-ray as the cause of hoareseness.

3. I gave ruta and arg.met on the basis of vocal cords (ligament) strain due to her being a teacher. The other homeopaths had given arnica which has no role in chronic ligament strain.

4. Voice rest, which of course other ENT surgeons have also advised.

It took six weeks before she became okay.

This treatment not only killed two birds with one stone but three birds since it cured her piles also which was due to chillies on which allopaths did not question since they were trying to be superspecialists

INNER EAR (Meniere's Disease)

Since the last edition of my book, large number of cases of Meniere's disease and Meniere's Syndrome, have come to me for homeopathic treatment when all allopathic treatment failed such as serc, stugeron, stametil, vertin.

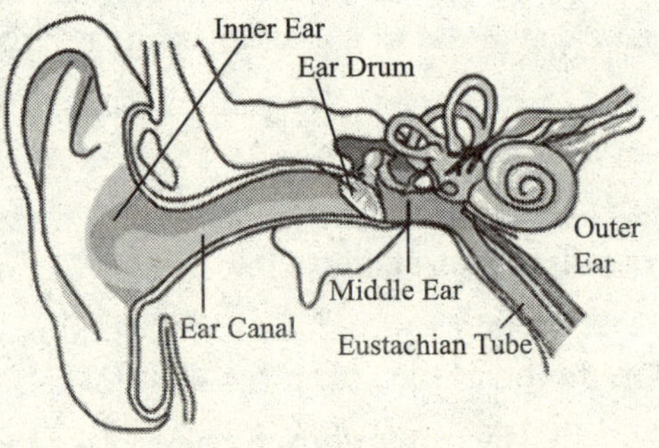

It is very essential to reassure such patients that there is nothing serious with their brain. The more their minds are fixated on noises or vertigo, the worst become their symptoms.

Homeopathy:

Apart from the treatment I have advised in my previous editions, I find the following treatment very beneficial in resistant cases of Meniere's disease.

1. Carboneum Sulphate 200 alternating with combination of coculus + Theridion.

In very elderly people, phosphorus and conium have been found to be of immense benefit.

Coculus and phosphorus take away the fear element, often associated in elderly people as if there is something sinister condition in the brain.

Inner Ear Deafness (Presbyacusis):

There is no treatment for sensor neural loss in old age.This is usually called Presbyacusis.

Homeopathy:

Case-1:

72-year-old man came asking treatment for his enlarged prostrate. So apart from sabal serrulata, I gave him Ferrum Picric and Kali mur 6x. He said, of course I do not think you can do anything for my old age deafness. After examining his ears, when I knew the cause, I gave the above treatment and to my surprise he told me he had immense improvement in his hearing as well in urine problem.

◆◆◆

5.

GASTROINTESTINAL

GASTRITIS (Acidity)

This is an extremely common condition, it is essential to understand its common causes before one can treat these cases.

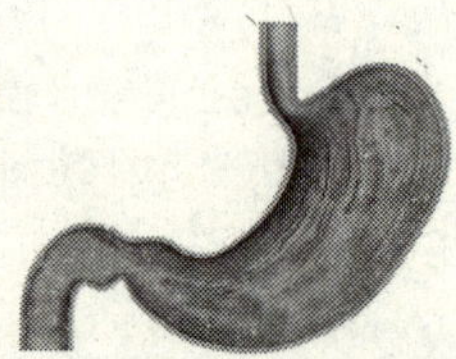

Gastritis (Acidity)

Causes:

1. Spicy food, irregular timings and overeating are the commonest causes of gastritis.
2. Alcohol, smoking, consuming excessive tea and coffee.
3. Allopathic medicines, most of them cause gastritis, sooner or later.
4. Emotional resentment, internal mental conflicts, anger.

Treatment:

I have seen thousands of patients being treated for the above condition after repeated endoscopy and getting the video-film to impress these patients.

Then they take the aspiration to make a diagnosis of H.pylori or take the biopsy to exclude malignancy.

Allopathy:

Most of these patients are put on Rabeprazole or Omnaprazole type of preparations with zintec and loads of digene liquid.

If it is H.pylori, the patients are impressed with being prescribed kit(comprising, antibiotic, antacid and antibiotics).

ACT:(Author's comment and treatment):

I have seen hundreds of gastroenterologists giving the above preparations for years without advising the patients to avoid the above-mentioned causative factors.

Giving the above treatment for too long causes constipation and piles in the patients and make them patients of colitis and then go on to repeated Colonoscopy and then the treatment of colitis starts along with gastritis.

My request to such patients is to ask these so-called specialists:

Are there any side effects(immediate or late) of the treatment being given to them?

It is their birthright to ask the doctor for such adverse effects.

Homeopathy:

Acid Reflux: Iris versicola, asfoetida, carboveg, abies nigra.

Gastritis: nux vomica and robinia and capsicum

Gastritis due to emotional stress such as near exams or husband wife argument or illness of near and dear ones–anacardium and ignatia.

ULCERATIVE COLITIS
(Irritable Bowel Syndrome)

I have dealt with this condition briefly even in my previous edition – however in view of the fact that patients are coming to me at incurable stage and with complications, thus in this edition I am writing a different line of treatment for the basic condition and also the treatment of complicated cases of ulcerative colitis.

It is essential to know the common causes of ulcerative colitis as given below:

1. Stress and strain of long standing etiology – whether professional, domestic or otherwise.
2. Spicy food especially red chillies and low roughage diet.
3. Strong allopathic drugs especially NSAID preparations, (combiflam, advil, brufen, voveran, diclogesic).
4. Metrogyl related drugs given often for amoebic colitis, given repeatedly or for prolonged periods itself cause aseptic colitis.
5. Strong antibiotics, including antitubercular drugs.

Irritable bowel syndrome is the precursor of colitis and ulcerative colitis. The common symptoms are constipation alternating diarrhoea.

In colitis, there is tenesmus, mucus, undigested stools, leading to weakness and emaciation.

Allopathy:

The common medicines given are salazine, colospa and in severe cases, steroids.

The side effects of these drugs are well-known to the public and patients are helpless to take it.

Homeopathy:

In my experience, dealing with thousands of such cases the following treatment is of unquestionable value.

However, those who had been on steroids, are more difficult to treat since they come with the side-effects of steroids(as mentioned in the previous book).

Ulcerative colitis patients with bleeding and lot of mucus needs the help of remedies like blumia, phosphorus and merc cor.

Ulcerative colitis due to stress and strain respond very satisfactorily to Anacardium, ignatia and kaliphos.

Radical change in the type of diet is a must in consultation with dietitian.

Author's Comments:

I feel in all the spoiled cases, patients are to be equally blamed since they never bothered to ask the doctor the side effects of medicines which they have been prescribed.

Moreover, these patients are very happy with repeated colonoscopies for their satisfaction that it is not cancer and satisfaction of the doctor since these investigation add to his pocket.

One or occasionally two endoscopies are sufficient but repeated without any clinical indication; I feel it is not justified.

PILES (Anal Fissure, Anal Fistula)

I have seen hundreds of such patients suffering from different degrees of severity. These are bleeding or non-bleeding piles. 50% of cases have come after having been operated upon and haemorrhoids have recurred again.

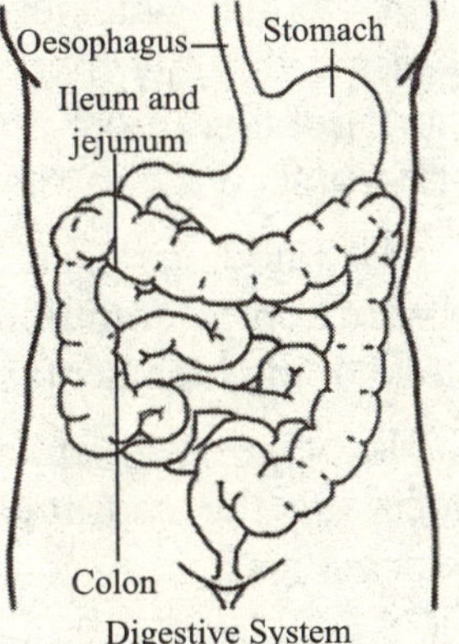

Digestive System

The common causes of piles are constipation, especially non-veg diet, with no roughage, or allopathic drugs especially antibiotics.

In Eastern countries, spicy food is the commonest cause of piles.

Allopathy:

The operation is not a permanent treatment; it is done either by injecting sclerosing agents into veins or operation.

Dafflon capsules are given to control bleeding but this can cause severe acidity.

Homeopathy:

I find the following remedies have miraculous results, provided the combinations of these are done in a scientific and synergistic effect with complement effect of remedies of each other.

I make the combinations according to individual's piles condition.

The remedies are following:

Nitric, ratanhea, aesculus, hammamelis, podophyllum and calcarea fluor. Locally I apply homeopathic cream and not allopathic anovate since anovate is simply local anaesthetic effect and masks the symptoms and does not cure the disease.

PANCREATITIS

I wonder whether gallbladder laproscopic surgeons are realising the fact that since laproscopic surgery is becoming more popular, more and more cases of pancreatitis (subacute or chronic) are becoming common.

MRI findings in such cases often reveal that there is some obstruction to common bile duct or due to slipping of stone while doing laproscopy.

In other cases, stricture of bile ducts are the causative factor of pancreatitis.

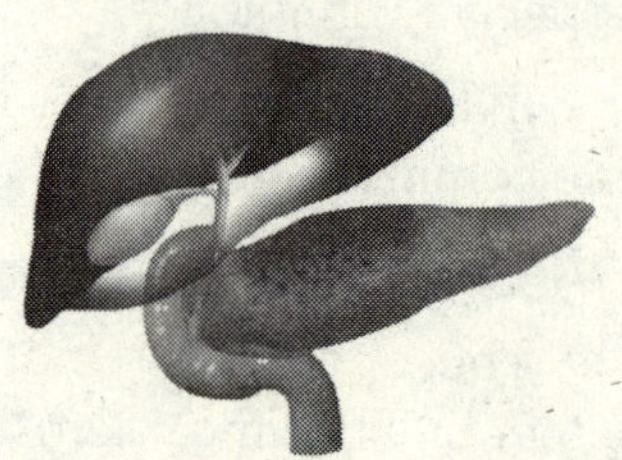

I have to deal with certain cases of pancreatic cysts after certain botch surgeries.

These cases have undergone repeatedly for stent insertions.

Homeopathy:

I have dealt such cases without any hope, and to my surprise, good results.

Iris versicola, iodum and phosphorus have given excellent results.

In cases of strictures, my aetiopathological treatment with calcarea fl. and clematis has given very good results.

◆◆◆

6.

LOCOMOTOR DISEASES

CERVICAL SPONDYLOSIS

This is a home word these days and the condition and its treatment though mentioned in my last edition, but more complicated cases had come to me since computer profession, call centre syndrome, wrong trainers in gyms have contributed to increased incidence of this disease.

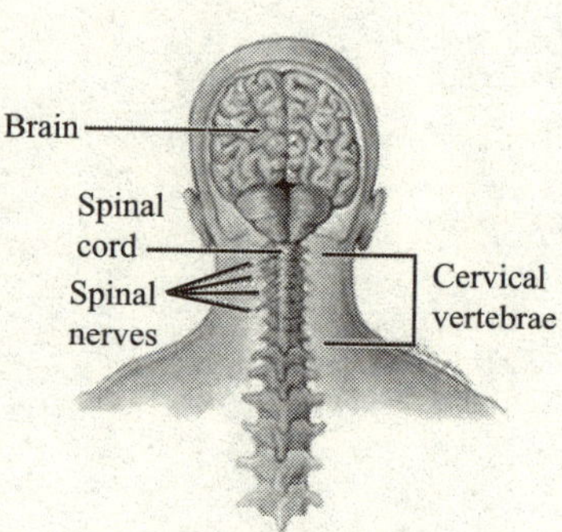

Cervical Spondylosis

Allopathy:

The common treatment is the painkillers which are often prescribed in increasing dosage or stronger ones.

The common side effects are gastritis, skin allergy or asthmatic attacks.

To counteract these side effects, they prescribe antiallergics which cause extreme dryness of skin making them permanent customers of the dermatologists.

Everybody is familiar with symptoms of cervical spondylosis, with referred pain to chest, arm and head, which can frighten the patient and can call for the opinion of cardiologist, neurologist, orthopaedic surgeon.

Once the diagnosis is established of cervical spondylosis, the treatment is the same in the hands of all allopathic specialists.

All the painkillers or medicines given for vertigo are not without side-effects.

However, physiotherapy in expert hands is an essential part of treatment, whether one takes homeopathy or allopathy.

Homeopathy:

I have to give different combinations in different groups, different potencies, in cyclic rotation, which control the vertigo also which in some cases is very frightening. The common remedies prescribed are:

Cimcifuga, causticum, rhus tox and calcarea fluor.

However, in severe pain instead of high potency of mag. phos, it is better to give in combination with other complementary medicines.

In some cases, where all allopathic medicines have failed, I have seen calcarea phos and gelsemium had a magic effect.

LOW BACKACHE (LUMBAGO)

This is one of the commonest conditions all over the world.

As an allopath and homeopath, practising both pathies, depending upon the type of case, personality, I have come to conclusion that for lumbago, it is much easier to treat with allopathy than with homeopathy.

Allopathy:

To prescribe painkillers, irrespective of the cause of lumbago is very easy. It is pity that patients do not ask the doctor the long-term side-effects of these medicines (combiflam, advil, flexon, mobizox). Often these have to be prescribed for a long time, then the side-effects make their appearance, as I mentioned in earlier chapters.

In resistant cases, in localised pain, the orthopaedic surgeon gives steroid injection (medrol in India and medrone in UK).

Patient feels quite happy in the beginning, but having knowledge of both the branches of medicine, steroid injection make future treatment with allopathy or homeopathy more difficult.

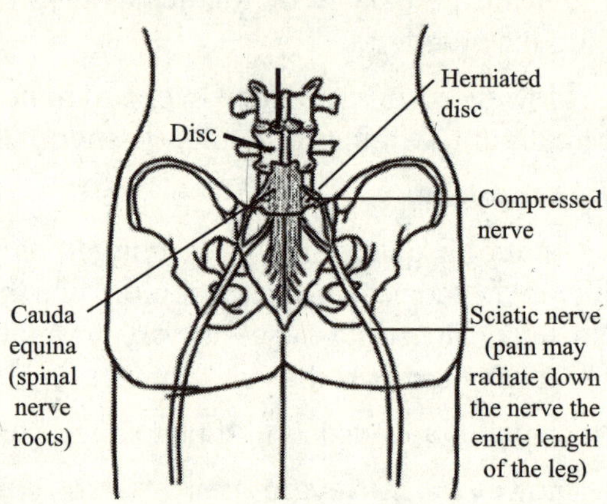

Homeopathy:

It is tailor-made as will be evident in the forthcoming homeopathic treatment:

In Women:

It is very common after EPIDURAL anaesthesia for caesarian operation. The condition is common because caesarian has become popular with gynae obst and with sophisticated women with sedentary lifestyle.

LEDUM PAL: is the remedy of choice in the experience of author.

Other homeo remedies in such cases cannot be equally effective. As to why this remedy, I think, homeopath would know my reasoning of prescribing it.

After Delivery:

The backache occurring after delivery Kalicarb is remedy of choice but one should not repeat it often and T.B. should be excluded before prescribing.

SEPIA is another remedy for women's backache, especially if it is associated with leucorrhoea and woman is of sensitive nature.

If you gave calcarea phos in addition to sepia, the woman would not need to be sent repeatedly to please the bone density protagonists.

In Men:

Never forget Rhus tox and ruta. Rhus tox must be given in high potencies, repeated at weekly intervals.

If there is associated piles, you can save the money of the patient by not sending to surgeon who will further complicate the case.

AESCULUS will work like a magic. It will kill two birds with one stone. It will cure low backache as well as piles.

MUSCULO-SKELETAL DISORDERS

ARTHRITIS

Here I will be dealing with two types of arthritis, i.e., osteoarthritis which is often due to ageing process, due to wear and tear of the joints or due to old injury.

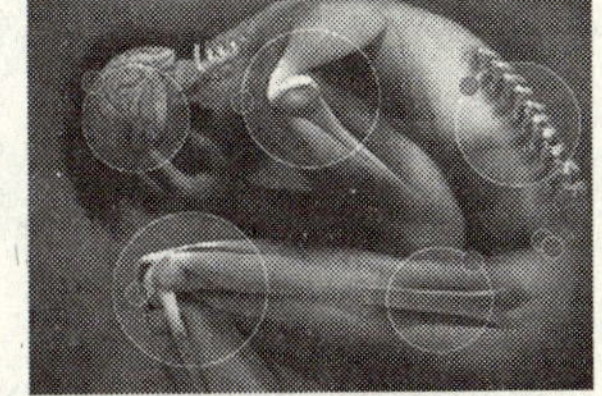

Musculo-Skeletal disorders Arthritis

The other which is more crippling and resistant to modern treatment is rheumatoid arthritis.

I am excluding rheumatic arthritis which is often seen in younger people, affecting mostly patients of poor socio-economic status who are prone to throat and dental infections.

OSTEOARTHRITIS

Despite the advances in knee and hip replacement, still lots of problems come to treat such patients.

Allopathy:

Every patient is not suitable for surgery owing to various other ailments such as diabetes, high blood pressure, heart condition.

The patients who had come to me after those surgeries were still taking painkillers as they were before surgery. During and immediate postoperatively lot of these patients are put on strong anti-inflammatory medication, which have caused serious side effects, such as kidney disturbances, erythema nodosum and severe gastritis and deep venous thrombosis and some cases of pulmonary embolism. Apart from these immediate and late complications, not all cases are successful.

Even the conservative treatment by allopathy is as dangerous as the surgery itself.

Many patients do not know the side effects of these anti-inflammatory drugs which I want to highlight and make them aware of. I will come to those dangerous side and toxic effects after the chapter of Rheumatoid Arthritis.

RHEUMATOID ARTHRITIS

I have seen patients are very happy if RA factor is negative in the blood report, however even with negative RA factor the disease is very crippling leading to marked disability in later stages.

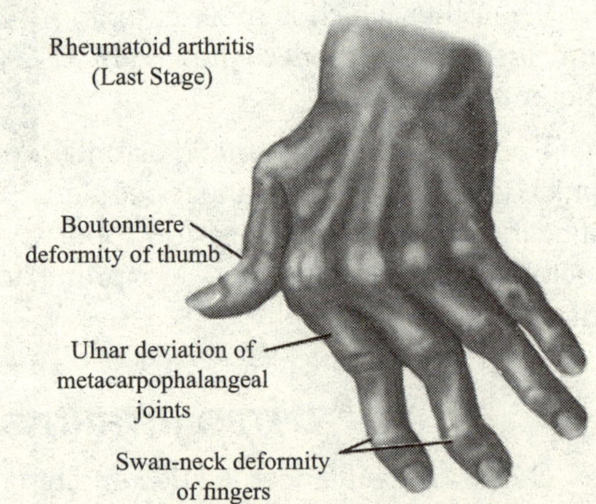

Leave alone the general physicians, even, so to say who call themselves Super-specialists or Rheumatologists and Immunologists, they make the condition of such patients worse with the side effects of strong allopathic medications than the disease itself.

Out of hundreds of such patients who came to see me after the side effects of allopathic medications were unbearable. I will quote two specimen cases with multiple side-effects, after having been treated by top Rheumatologists in Mumbai and Delhi.

Case-1:

A man of 45 years from Baroda came to see me with the following multiple side effects with the original disease still persisting.

The story goes like this: He went to a physician with complaints of pain and stiffness in limbs. As usual, he was put on NSAID preparations (Brufen, Diclofenac and Aspirin). He developed mouth ulcers and gastritis for which he was given antacids. Then he was referred to rheumatologist who put him on Methotrexate once a week. The patient was happy in the beginning but soon became resistant to treatment.

Then he was put on Chloraquin along with Methotrexate. This patient was waiting for my return from U.K. where I had gone for an important assignment.

Now the patient had multiple problems when he came to see me. His symptoms now were:

A. Breathlessness on slight exertion, cough and chest pain.

B. Gastric pain and Diarrhoea.

C. Skin pigmentation lichen planus.

D. Extreme weakness.

All the above symptoms were due to side effects of Methotrexate.

The most disappointing thing was that when he was sent to the topmost chest physician of Delhi because of chest symptoms, he put him on anti-tubercular treatment (ATT) for 3 months, without any relief. It is a pity that chest physician did not bother to read a few lines in British National formulary to know the side effects of Methotrexate.

The patient developed eye complications due to ATT.

For gastric symptoms, he had been subjected to gastroscopy and then put on antacid.

With above complications developing, the patient's arthritic pain had gone to the background.

He was looking 65-year-old instead of 45. It took me six months to cure this patient.

Homeopathy:

1. For eyes and lungs: I gave Phosphorus
2. For skin complications: I gave combination of Arsenic iod and Apis.
3. For liver: I gave Jondila
4. For joint pains & stiffness: I gave combination of cal. Fluor+ causticum+ ruta

The above remedies would not have worked without giving Medorrhanium and Thuja at high potencies in between.

Case-2:

Allopathy:

A middle-aged lady came after having latest treatment from Army Hospital Rheumatologist. Apart from getting better, her rheumatic condition was worse than before because she had added other ailments on the top of Arthritis because of toxic and side effects of modern painkillers.

She was first put on NSAID preparations (Brufen) despite being given antacids. Then she was put on Vioxx, it was not banned at that time, she developed Angina.

Due to NSAID preparations, she developed severe psoriasis for which she was being given steroids preparations, which caused complications like facial hair, high blood pressure.

Homeopathy:

I started treatment by giving Medorrhanium 1M as there was history of persistent vaginal discharge a few years ago for which she was given allopathic treatment.

Then I gave her Rhus tox and Natrum sulphate potencies alternating with each other.

Her fluid retention due to steroid got better with nat. sulphate, Rhus tox looked after arthritis and psoriasis. In between I had to give her high potency of Thuja 1M since all her troubles started after she was given tetanus vaccine during pregnancy.

Then I had to give her Apis to get rid of her fluid retention and remaining rashes on her body which occurred due to Brufen.

The most regrettable thing is patients come for homeopathic treatment very late with half-hearted faith and come at a stage not only with the original disease, but other ailments which have already occurred due to allopathic drugs' side effects.

Another new drug Prosigesic one of the Cox-2 inhibitor has to be suddenly banned because of its side effect on the liver.

I fail to understand how many drugs take a sudden U-turn in, so-called scientifically proved drugs in allopathy.

◆◆◆

7.
TUMOURS

MODEL CURE

Here in this chapter, I am dealing with benign tumours which are not easily amenable to treatment.

Lipomas, Fibrolipomas Non-Hodgkin Lymphomas.

LIPOMAS, FIBROLIPOMAS

Case-1:

These tumours are becoming very common owing to the increase in number of vaccinations than what it used to be 20 years ago.

Allopathy:

Every surgeon knows at heart that even after radical surgery, these are notorious for recurrence. As a result patients are reluctant to undergo surgery, unless the tumours are unsightly or causing a bit of discomfort or pain.

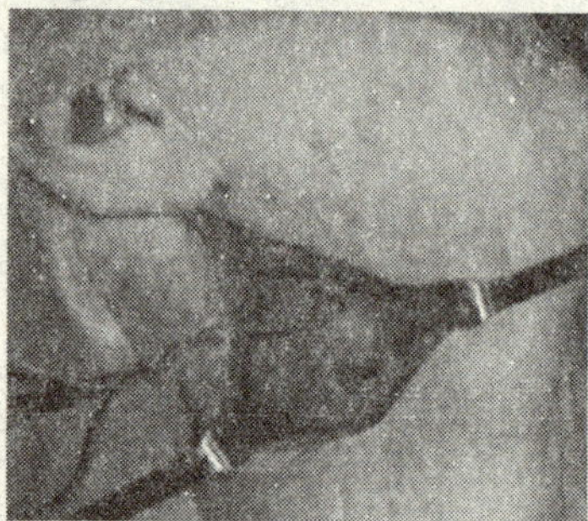

Lipomas

Homeopathy:

I reluctantly took two cases without any hope or assurance to the patient.

One was a young man of 35 years, from middle-east with multiple fibrolipoma. After giving high potence of thuja, this was followed by the following combination:

Baryta carb, calcarea iodide, conium. To my surprise, he responded in 2 weeks time. The tumours became softer. Then I ommited calc. iodide and conium and put him on calcarea carb and baryta carb. This satisfied customer brought a friend of his with soft Lipomas.

Case-2:

The second patient of lipoma I treated with only calcarea carb and baryta carb.

LYMPHANGIOMA

Case-1

This child of 3 years, had lymphangioma in left submandibular region.

The surgery was fraught with danger owing to the danger of mandibular division of facial nerve. The second reason for reluctance to get operated upon was that it was likely to recur and not always easy to remove in toto.

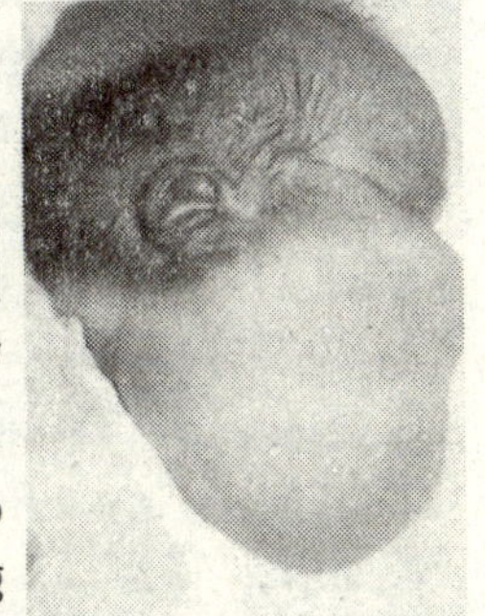

Lymphangioma

As the tumour was not present at birth and developed a few months after BCG and triple vaccination, I gave thuja, followed by calcarea carb and hammamelis.

It took three months for the tumour to recede to 50% and at the time of writing his case history, the treatment is being continued.

ACT(Author's comments and treatment): Most of the allopaths label these as autoimmune diseases. The cause of this disturbance of immunity is our strong allopathic treatment such as steroids given for allergy (skin or chest) which itself is caused by these vaccinations (read chapter on vaccinations in 3rd edition of my book 'Homeopathy Cures Where Allopathy Fails').

CYSTS, BUMPS AND LUMPS

These conditions are becoming very common these days, leading to anxiety and fear amongst the sufferers in case it is the word C.

That fear leads to so many unnecessary investigations and unnecessary surgery and after keeping update with health in West and East, this will eventually lead to bankruptcy of NHS in West and Poverty to common man by greedy doctors in the East.

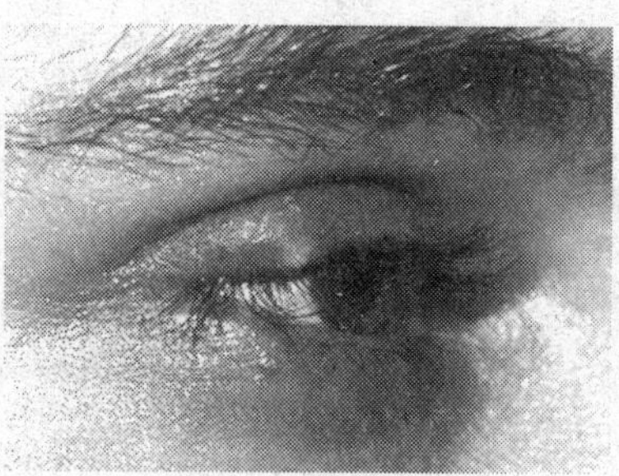

Cysts, bumps and lumps

The patient when noticing these things get panicky and obsessional, as a result doctors in the West to guard themselves against medico-legal cases of negligence lead to this course of action.

Following are the common tumours, which to the clinical sense of a good clinician should not lead to unnecessary investigations or to go under the knife.

1. *Bunions:* Usually hard bony prominence along the base of big toe, it is often due to wrong fitting or too pointed sole shoes.

   So the treatment lies in wearing proper shoes.

2. *Cysts:* These are fluid filled bags around back of knees or at the elbow, called housemaid knees or tennis elbow. These are due to continuous friction or excessive friction

of synovial membranes which act as shock absorber normally.

The best treatment is to avoid the causative factor.

3. *Ganglion:* These are usually at the back of joints, commonly at the back of wrist. These are notorious for recurrences.
4. *Lipomas:* These are soft mobile tumours, can be on any part of body, usually painless and can be multiple. Notorious for recurrences.
5. *Chalazion:* It is firm tumour in any of eyelids, can be single or multiple.

Treatment:

Allopathy:

Surgery is the only treatment, but as I mentioned that in all cases, recurrence of the tumour is a rule rather than exception.

Homeopathy:

1. *Bunion:* Avoid the causative factor.
2. *Ant.:* Crudum 200 is the remedy of choice.
3. *Cysts:* Apis +bell. are often successful.
4. *Ganglion:* Acid benzoic and Ruta in high potencies are very good remedies.
5. *Chalazion:* Calcarea fluor and acid nitric in higher and higher potencies are excellent.
6. *Lipomas:* Baryta carb and conium in selective potencies, depending upon the experience of homeopath.

Lumps in breast in women especially in very young girls.

◆◆◆

8.

GYNAECOLOGICAL DISEASES

VAGINITIS AND LEUCORRHOEA

This inflammation of vagina whether bacterial or fungal or both, every third woman gets in life at one or the other stage in life.

The unfortunate thing they do not realise, neither my gynae, obs. colleagues realise that vaginitis causes cystitis and cystitis cause vaginitis.

Treating cystitis with antibiotics leads to side effect of fungal infection.

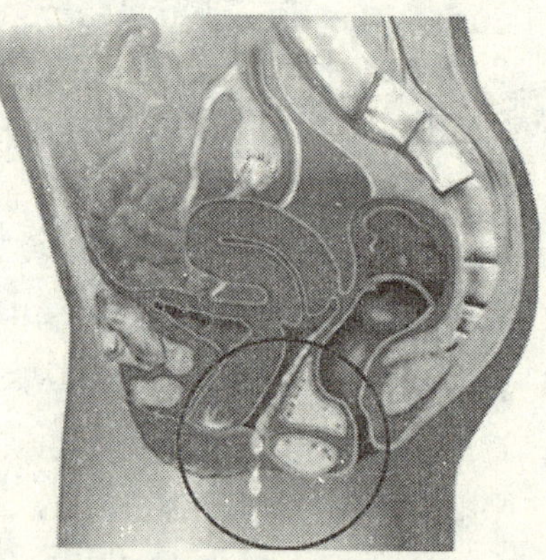

Vaginitis and Leucorrhoea

To cure completely, one must clear cystitis and vaginitis completely rather than for cystitis sending to urologist and for vaginitis sending to gyna/obs. Each one deals in their own way, leaving one organ affected.

Homeopathy:

Severe resistant cases of vaginitis and leucorrohoea, I have seen responding very well to eupionum, apart from kalibio.

It is essential to rule out other focus of infection like sinusitis in the body.

The second important thing I wish to bring home to the patient, lactobacill acidophilus must be taken whenever antibiotics are prescribed to prevent fungal infection.

REGARDING RECURRENT CYSTITIS

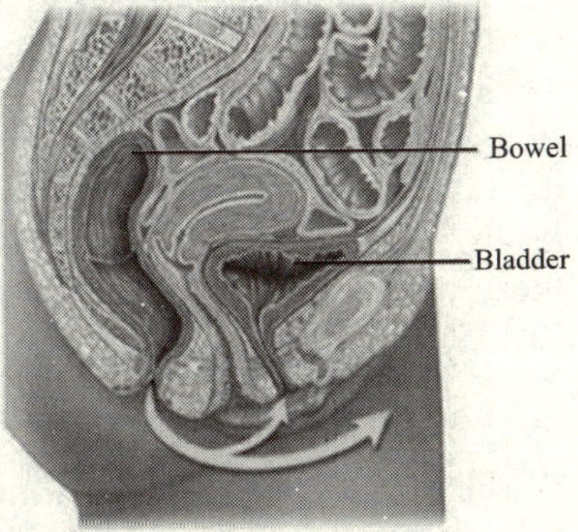

In my experience, repeated courses of broadspectrum antibiotics, even according to culture and sensitivity,have failed to prevent recurrent infection. The immunity of the patient further goes down with antibiotics, apart from the fact these encourage fungal infection as side effect.

My prescription for recurrent urinary infection in women mentioned in the kidney chapter has never failed me. It is a golden prescription.

POLYCYSTIC OVARIES SYNDROME (PCOS)

I have written quite a few chapters on polycystic ovaries and as I mentioned the incidence of its occurrence is on the rise.

The allopaths say the exact cause is not known or probably is genetic. This is the common excuse on the part of allopaths.

In my experience, the reason for rise in incidence is due to allopathic treatment of slight irregular periods which is common these days owing to stress and strain of life.

Stress and strain affect hormones through hypothalamus.

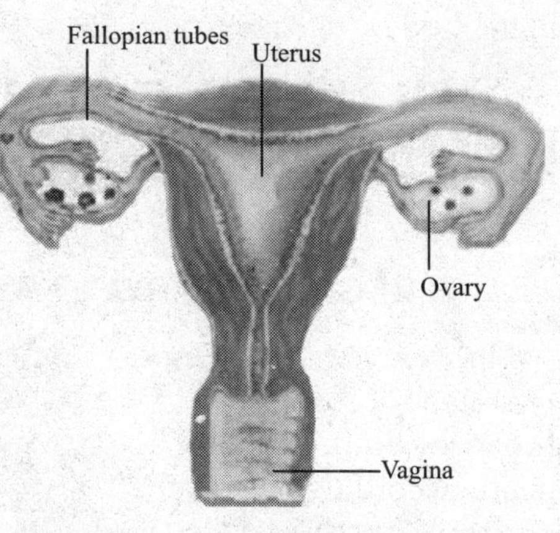

To regulate the periods, the obs. and gyne. surgeons give hormonal preparations which lead to polycystic ovaries since these artificial hormones stimulate the ovaries to pharmacological levels. By causing these polycystic ovaries, often the following symptoms are of PCOS.

1. Lack of ovulation for an extended period of time.
2. High levels of male hormones (androgens).
3. Hirsutism(excessive growth of facial hair).
4. Diminution of breast size.
5. Infertility.
6. Acanthosis nigricans(darkened skin areas on the back of neck, in the armpits, under the breast).
7. Symptoms of hypothyroidism (excessive weight, constipation, etc).

Allopathy:

There is no satisfactory solution except removing the cysts or giving various hormones which further endanger the malignancy of breast.

Homeopathy:

Examination is a must especially in married women.

Ultrasound is also very helpful to confirm the diagnosis.

Thuja is the main remedy.

Calcarea carb is of immense value if the ovarian cyst is associated with heavy periods and woman is obese and of fair complexion.

My combination of the following remedies have never let me down:

Apis, bell, cimcifuga, colocynth, arnica.

MENSTRUAL PROBLEMS

Amenorrhoea

Secondary amenorrhoea: late menses, scanty menses, irregular menses are creating problems in epidemic proportions.

The cases are spoilt because of allopathic treatment, since that involves giving hormones, usually the gynaecologists say at the commencement, that it is for a short duration – which is the start of following complications caused by gynae-obstetricians although unintentionally. Even the educated patients do not bother to ask the gynaecologist whether it is permanent treatment and are there any side effects of long-term medication.

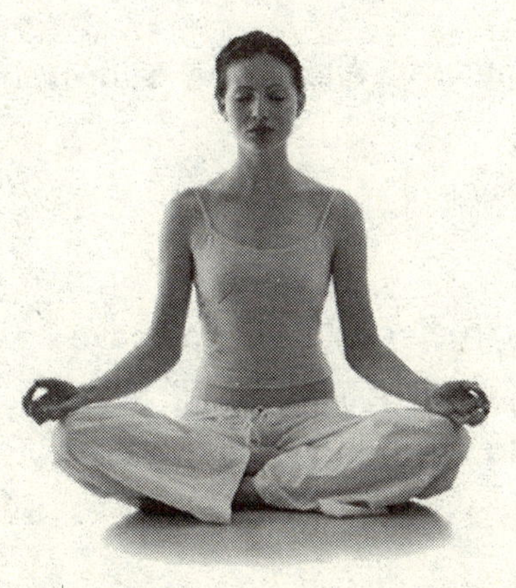

The following case gives a very good picture of what happens with hormonal treatment.

Case 1 & 2:

Two young stunning beauties, both being allopathic doctors qualified 2 years ago, married to doctors, who were settled in USA, believed strongly in allopathic treatment.

Both had secondary amenorrhoea in the final year of M.B.B.S. They were treated by their Gynae Professor, and then by Endocrinologist of repute and Gynae. consultant, at a reputed hospital in Delhi. After 18 months treatment, they came to me when they had put on enormous weight and happened to read my book. Very few gynaecologists remember the basic physiology that hypothalamus controls the anterior pituitary which controls the thyroid and ovarian hormones. These specialists forget that this hormonal upset is due to the overactivity of hypothalamus because of stress and strain. These above-mentioned sisters started irregular periods due to the stress of final M.B.B.S. exams.

Although they were also put on alprax by the endocrinologist and Gynae. which made them drowsy and lethargic.

Homeopathy:

I put them on two combinations, alternating with each other.

A. Ignatia +Aurum met+kali phos

B. Cimcifuga+pulsatilla +sepia.

Lachesis once a week due to their constitutional make up.

Within four months their periods became regular. Water retention which occurred due to hormones was treated with nat. sulph and nat. mur.

PREMENSTRUAL TENSION SYNDROME

This is one of the commonest malady afflicting young girls since its inception. However, it is becoming more common and more severe in intensity owing to change in lifestyle and modern stresses and strain making the youngsters highly stung and nervous.

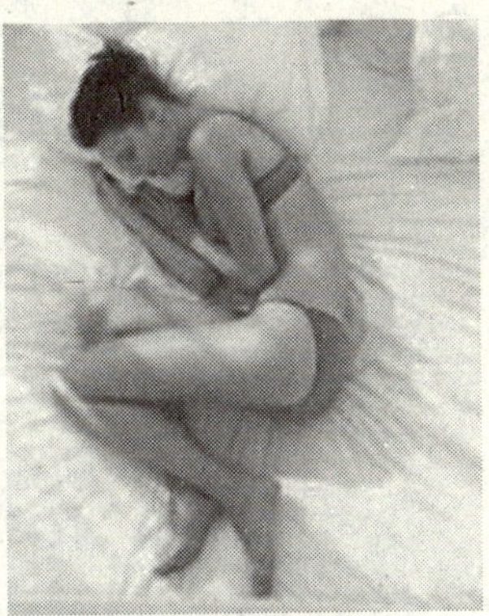

Premenstrual Tension Syndrome

The symptoms can range from mild to severe to the extent of epileptic fits or severe depression or even to the extent of suicide or homicide.

Allopathy:

Very simple for the gynae. They simply put them on tranquillisers and hormones so as to cause the following side effects:

1. Drowsiness and lethargy, which interferes with their studies.
2. Hormones like contraceptive pills, which lead to increase in weight and obesity, which further leads to inferiority complex, and finally lead to depression.
3. Then for depression they put on antidepressants which further cause obesity of enormous degree.

Homeopathy:

Most girls have come to me at this stage.

1. My combination of ignatia, aurum met and acid phos has controlled the major emotional symptoms like irritability and depression.

2. My antispasmodic mixture has controlled all sorts of spasmodic pain (mag.phos.+cyclamen=colocynth).
3. I have successfully controlled minor epilepsy due to premenstrual syndrome, along with violent temper by cicuta virosa.

Then I give medication to regularise and to have easy menses, with cimcifuga and pulsatilla.

MENOPAUSE HYSTERECTOMY AND OVARIECTOMY

These are the patients with worse symptoms of hormonal and emotional disturbances, especially who had unilateral or bilateral ophorectomies.

I have seen most Gynae-Obs. remove the ovaries giving the patients explanation of doing so that these are not serving any purpose by the time they are removed. But this is not correct in practical experience, going by the symptoms these women suffer after ablation of these organs. Another explanation given by the Gynae-Obs. is that these may not undergo malignant change; despite the fact the uterus is removed for benign fibroids rather than cancerous.

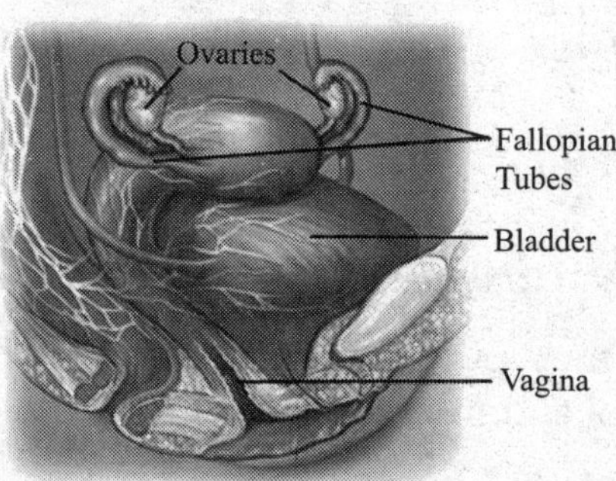

Symptoms:

Loss of libido is extreme in such cases. The other predominant symptom is extreme degree of nervousness in these women.

Allopathy:

The common treatment is to put them on hormones irrespective of the dangers of cancer of breast or stroke.

Antidepressants which lead to increase in weight and danger of gastric bleeding, if they are also taking Brufen for arthritis.

Homeopathy:

I find excellent results in these two distressing and debilitating symptoms by giving them:

Ooophorinum in trituration

Oxytropin in dilution controls the nervous symptoms like a magic.

For loss of libido following hysterectomy and removal of ovaries, my combination of crossmodium (high) and agnus c and sepia ampete viagra for men.

◆◆◆

9.

KIDNEY & URINARY PASSAGE DISEASES

URINARY
STRICTURE OF URETHRA

This is a condition where there is narrowing of the urinary passage, more common in males than females owing to narrow and long and tortuous urethra in contrast to straight and wide urethra in women.

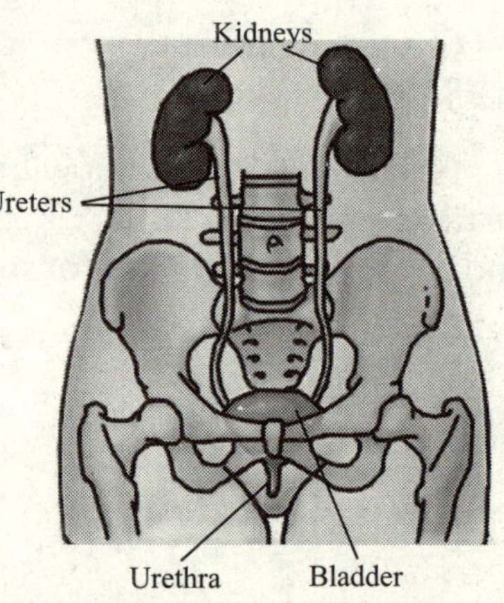

The condition is either congenital or acquired (accidental or surgically induced).

The following case which I took as a challenge proves my statement that homeopathy works where allopathy fails.

Case:

A young boy of 20 years with no history of any UTI infection had dilatation by urologist of repute in Delhi but the condition recurred. So he went to the topmost homeopath of international fame who was honest to tell the patient that he cannot offer anything since the cause is surgical.

So I took it as a challenge and put him on the following homeo medicines based treatment on the basic pathology of the disease that there is fibrosis and cicatrix and not mere spasm, this is leading to UTI infection which itself increases fibrosis—thus a vicious cycle sets up.

The patient had lots of warts on the neck. He had also stiffness of the back due to fibrosis.

I commenced my treatment with 1M dose of thuja followed by the following combinations of my cocktail:

A. Staph.200+clematis 200

B. Cal.fl.200+causticum200+thiosin30(to break the fibrosis and cicatrix)

He got 80% improvement in 7 days time.

However, I have warned him not to let the urine become acidic.

For his low backache, I gave him cim.+hypericum+ruta.

INTRACTABLE UTI

This was a challenging case of UTI in a 40-year-old lady doctor– a urologist herself who had intractable UTI for the last 5-6 years and had been having all the broad spectrum antibiotics but she had relief only for a short time when the infection used to recur after a few weeks. Repeated culture and antibiotics failed to control the infection permanently. I treated her with homeo. as below:

Homeopathy:

Firstly, I treated her vaginal fungal infection which was the cause for recurrence with lactobacil.

She had seen her gynae colleague for that who treated her with repeated antibiotics locally and internally, with the result that antibiotics further increased fungal infection. Due to proximity of vagina to urethral opening, the UTI used to recur.

The urine microscopy examination showed 80 to 100 pus cells.

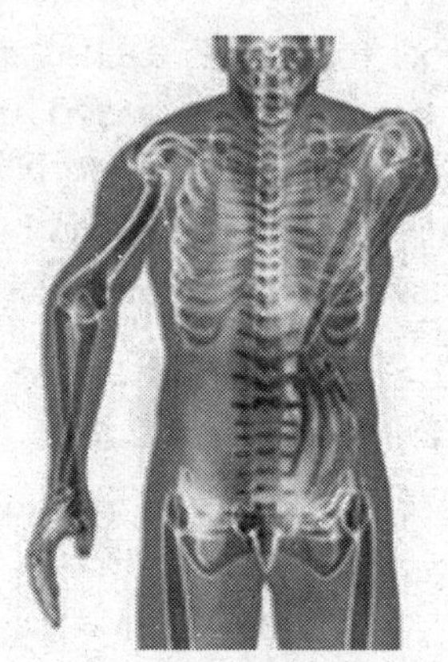

Intractable U.T.I.

I gave her cantharis, eupatorium.p and equeisteum and within a week, the urine examination was normal.

For her vaginal fungal infection, I gave her acid nitric, lactobacil.

However, I had excluded any infection in her husband.

She is a strong believer in homeopathy now.

◆◆◆

10.

NEUROLOGICAL DISEASES

MULTIPLE SCLEROSIS

This condition is characterised by numbness, weakness of lower limbs gradually progressing upwards. The other typical symptoms in many of my patients are vertigo (dizziness), blurring of vision and diplopia (seeing double).

The following cases will demonstrate that in most cases it is the allopathic treatment with its adverse effects that have caused M.S. (multiple sclerosis).

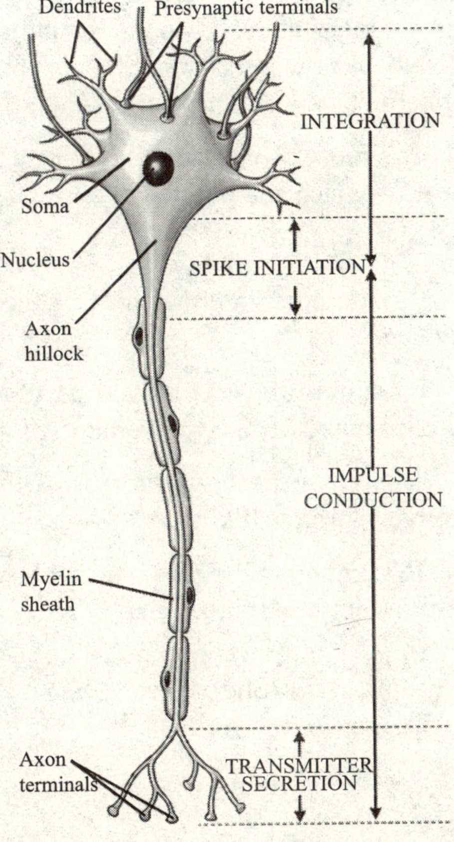

The worst thing is that allopathic treatment for M.S. is not only a complete failure but its treatment with steroids have caused so many other ailments before they came to me for its homeopathic treatment.

Case-1:

A young lady of 26 years came to me after being diagnosed with M.S. and having been treated at reputed private hospitals in Delhi with steroids, the only treatment available with allopaths anywhere in the world. She had three relapses within a period of 18 months. By this time, she got facial hairs, weakness of limbs. Blurring of vision and vertigo was still persisting. She also had gastric problems due to steroids and puffiness of face.

The cause of ailment in this patient was the recent treatment for acne which she had taken for two years.

Homeopathy:

I started treatment with Conium, as it was ascending paralysis.

Plumbum and oxalic acid as it was affecting the spinal cord. She had 50% improvement.

Then I replaced oxalic acid with lathyrus and she got dramatic improvement.

To counteract the side-effects of steroids I had to give her natrum mur and natrum sulph.

In six months, this girl was completely different than when she came to me. She was cheerful and 90% of M.S. symptoms were cured.

Case-2:

This case of M.S. was due to side effects of anti-tubercular treatment (ATT) which was stopped 3 months after its commencement since ATT was given not on confirmed diagnosis of T.B.

She went to U.S.A. for treatment of M.S. but after three courses of steroid treatment, she developed high BP and diabetes and came to me with steroid induced disease syndrome plus multiple sclerosis.

Homeopathy:

I commenced treatment with nitric acid (to counter the side-effect of strong antibiotics).

Then I gave Argentum nitrate and Oxalic acid for severe apprehension and very fond of sweets and severe post root pains respectively.

H1N1 — INFLUENZA VACCINE

Everybody is well aware and some people were in panic, more so in the West and during this epidemic I was in UK, and the public and hospital staff were in queue to get the vaccination done.

Those rich and resourceful in India were proud to get the vaccine from abroad. They had scant idea of possible side-effects of vaccine until they realised much later.

It is documented that Guillain-barre syndrome is one of the complication of the vaccine.

The clinical picture of guillain-barre syndrome is similar to multiple sclerosis, with particular emphasis is that in this syndrome the paralysis is ascending in nature, which is important from point of view of homeopathic treatment as it is different in descending type of paralysis.

As a prevention, I personally took homeo vaccine against

H1N1 virus and many of my patients who were against vaccine or could not get vaccine were treated with homeo vaccine.

I had a call from quite a few patients from abroad who took H1N1 vaccine, with side effects manifesting a few weeks after vaccination.

Seeing a couple of cases of guillain-barre syndrome after H1N1 vaccine, I was reminded when I had to do an emergency treachostomy on a young girl with guillain-barre (not of course due to H1N1 vaccine) in Cardiff some 30 years ago, since the paralysis was affecting respiratory muscles.

AUTISM, DOWN'S SYNDROME AND CEREBRAL PALSY

Most people must have noticed in the last few years, the above three diseases have gained epidemic proportions, especially in the West. The statistics show around 1 in 1000 child is suffering to a different severity from either of the illness.

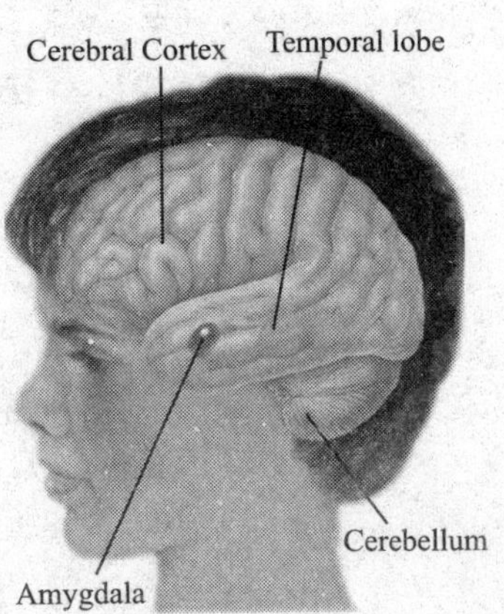

The other common illnesses manifesting a couple of years after birth are deafness with consequent speech deformity and optic atrophy.

Recently I had quite a few queries from Europe if there is anything that can be done with homeopathy. The answer is regrettably negative not because of the illness but because such patients come too late.

As it is often seen that they seek alternative treatment after exhausting all their resources, energies and time with most sophisticated investigations and referred to different specialists and super-specialists.

Allopathy:

The allopaths do not know the aetiology, hence do not know the treatment.

They can only suggest rehabilitation and no doubt, it is a long-term prison for the parents.

To blame genetics is an easy escape from ignorance of diagnosis as the probable cause.

Homeopathy:

People must be aware of the fact that lot of controversy has recently gone in debating as to whether MMR vaccine should be given or not since lot of cases of above syndromes have come into notice. Theories have been coming in favour of Dr. Wakefield in U.K. who has given statistics about the complications of this vaccine.

Admittedly, vaccines have revolutionised the positive outcome of illnesses since the discovery of first smallpox vaccine by Dr. Jenner in 1876.

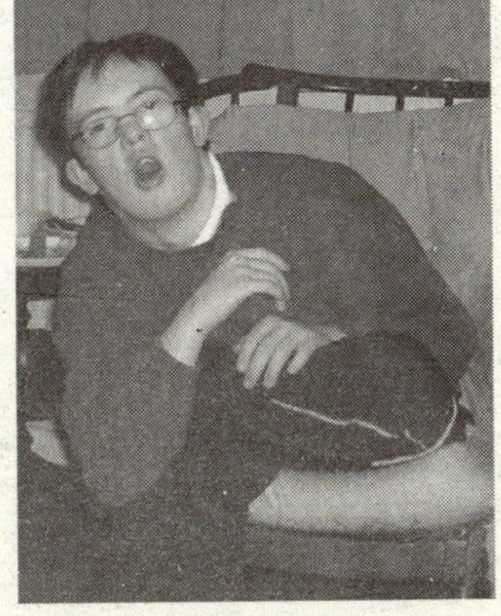

Most of the homeopaths are against vaccines, which I do not agree with their theories.

I feel vaccines should be given, but their side effects should be and can be prevented to a large extent by giving homeopathy at a proper time by an experienced homeopath.

I have dealt at length as to why the side effects of vaccines occur, in the last book 'Homeopathy Cures Where Allopathy Fails'.

Most of the diseases attributed to vaccines, though manifesting late, I have treated on the basis of above aetiology. To mention a few, I will say:

1. Migraine
2. Bronchial asthma
3. Eczema
4. Psoriasis
5. Rheumatoid arthritis

◆◆◆

11.

EMOTIONAL DISEASES

These diseases are gaining epidemic proportions in all age groups.

I will deal each age group separately since aetiology is different in each age group.

A. *Genetic factor(Hereditary):* is no doubt quite common cause in all age groups.

Often parents who are high strung and hypersensitive have often offsprings of an emotional nature

B. *Acquired:* In Children, this is one of the common causes.

This has a lot of bearing on the emotional outcome of present day children.

Under acquired aetiology, I would subtitle them as under:

a. Fights amongst parents lead to conflicts in children's minds and they find an easy path out of the two opinions of the parents, irrespective of the result of his decision

b. Peer pressure

c. Riches, T.V., mobile, internet and magazines: are also responsible for the spoiled present day children.

d. Law against corporal punishment without the lawmakers realise that you cannot apply the same stick to everybody. Each case has to be dealt accordingly. Most educationists have followed the West and as a result the crime amongst children in India is growing with the same speed as in the West.

The old principle still holds good 'Spare the rod, spoil the child'. In olden times, we have never heard of children murdering their parents.

The percentage of children who are very sensitive in nature and need careful handling are only a few.

In Adolescents: The conflict between the emerging sexual emotions of subconscious mind and discipline (imaginary or real) of parents and society leads to a lot of crime, depression, hatred, suicide and homicide and uncontrollable anger.

Imbalance and conflict of these emotions are the commonest of present day crime amongst children of today.

Allopathy:

Tranquillisers and antidepressants are the only treatment which has its side effects of dependence, addiction and obesity, thyroid affection.

The patients are incapacitated with these drugs since it makes them drowsy and lethargic.

Homeopathy:

a. Psychotherapy (Introspection and realising the origin of these emotions).

b. For Anger: Chamomilla, Staphysagaria, Belladonna are the mainstay.

c. In schizophrenia cases, strammonium and hyoscyamus are the main line of treatment.

d. Religious mania should be routed out.

e. For depression, ignatia and aurum met after natrum mur is usually successful.

f. In some severe cases, I had given with tarantula his.

g. Proper teaching on sex.

OBSESSIVE COMPULSIVE DISORDER (OCD)

This condition is unfortunately very crippling and common amongst young and middle-aged people.

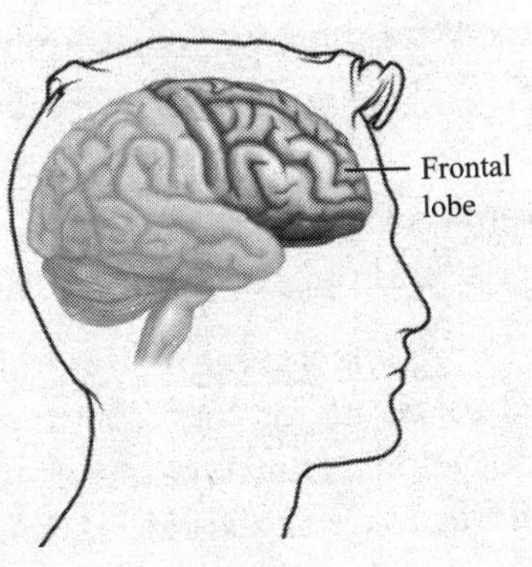

Aetiology:

It is difficult to draw the boundaries between discipline and indiscipline, freedom and inhibition. Consequently, there is an internal conflict in mind between two opposing forces (conscious and unconscious). In short, subconscious mind desires something, while conscious mind tries to control those desires.

A. Strict discipline, parents enforcing rigid rules and sex taboos at impressionable age is the common cause of OCD in the Asian countries.

B. In the West, cancer phobia created by media and so-called health awareness advocates going too far leading to anxiety, neurosis, cardiac neurosis and cancer phobia and obsession fears in public.

One does not realise as to how many diseases are created by these overenthusiastic doctors and media. Public should be careful in accepting blindly what these health educators say, realising that every week their theories and research results take a U-turn. All the investigations done to give assurance to these patients fail to give satisfaction, as exemplified in one of the following patients out of hundreds patients seen.

Case-1:

A 20-year-old girl had read in a female's magazine about cancer of breast and emphasis on mammography and other investigations. The girl got so severe phobia about cancer of the breast that she was examining her breast whole day in the mirror for any sign of cancer.

The gynaecologists did all the investigations and examination and reassured her there is nothing wrong with her breast and put her on tranquilliser.

The patient came to me through one of my satisfied customers and asked me as to: 'Why the lady doctor has put her on this medication if I have no cancer. It means there is something wrong with me and the obstetrician wants to hide it from me.'

Treatment:

Allopathy:

This girl was very brilliant and gold medallist until a few years ago, when she suffered from OCD which crippled her mentally and physically. The tranquillisers prescribed by the psychiatrists, neurologists and Gynae., obs. were making her drowsy all the time, as a result her grade started going down.

Homeopathy:

I started treatment with Syphllinum 1M and then after 2 days I gave her following two combinations:

A. Ignatia +Aurum met (contradiction and depression)

B. Anacardium +acid phos. (Conflict in mind + emotions affecting physically)

She was cheerful for 2 weeks then again got fear in her mind, in case she has got something in the head.

Then I gave Nat. mur 1M (chronic of Ignatia), she improved a lot after nat. mur and was okay for six weeks when she happened to read another magazine which frightened her to death, in case she has got brain tumour and is going mad. The MRI of brain did not reveal anything.

With this symptom, I gave Calcarea carb followed by 2 days later, Ancardium morning and kali phos. at night.

She was very introverted and at such an adult age lost all the interest in opposite sex. I gave Lycopodium 1M followed by 2 days later Agnus. C and she gradually recovered to a normal cheerful girl.

Conclusively, homeopathy with counselling is the safest and permanent line of treatment. It requires patience from both sides (patient and doctor).

MENTAL ILLNESSES

Allopathy:

Most of the antidepressants lead to increase in weight, drug dependence and habit forming. Because of increase in weight these patients further go into depression.

Homeopathy:

The following case histories will clearly demonstrate the results of homeopathy.

Case-1:

A young lady of 27 years was brought to me in Delhi from England with severe depression.

She had one broken affair and another broken marriage. She had all the modern allopathic treatment in U.K. without any long-term benefit. All she got was either drowsiness or state of exhalations from allopathy. Physically she became a skeleton, very short-tempered, now lost interest in opposite sex, venting her anger on her father. She had lost sleep and appetite since stopping allopathic medicines. In short, she was having withdrawal symptoms of allopathic antidepressants.

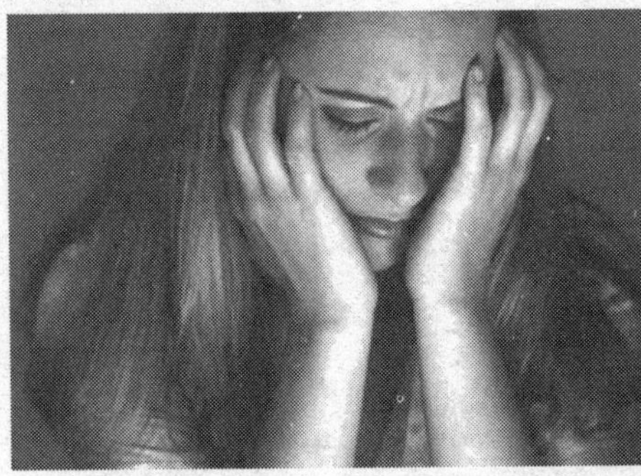

Showing Mental Illness

I started treatment with single dose of Natrum Mur10M (chronic of ignatia).Three days after taking nat. mur, her father said he noticed a smile on her face for the first time after five years. Two weeks later, she went into relapse with depression again. Then I gave her combination of Ignatia and Aurum met. in increasing potencies. She improved in appetite, started taking interest in opposite sex and other worldly affairs. She started having sound sleep. After a month, she again went into relapse, and then I gave her conium 1M on the basis of sexual frustration. Again, she started taking interest in opposite sex. She was a changed person for 2 months and then again went into depressive phase. Then I gave her Lycopodium 1M because of her introverted nature. Two days after lycopodium, I gave her acid phos. 200 and then onwards she became a cheerful girl taking interest in opposite sex. And now she is happily married in U.K.

Case-2:

A very obese girl was suffering from severe depression since the birth of her child. She became obese after taking antidepressants. According to her photograph, she was a skinny girl before the antidepressants. With antidepressants, her married life also got affected. I started the treatment with Thuja 1M, as she had three tetanus vaccines during pregnancies. Then I started treatment with homeo-thyroid as she had developed hypothyroid due to antidepressants.

Another cause of her obesity was that she was given hormones for scanty periods. Her scanty periods were due to depression as her hormonal essay was normal.

For her amenorrhoea, I gave combination of pulsatilla, sepia and cimcifuga.

Now she is a cheerful lady, has started taking interest in her child and has conceived again.

HOMEOPATHIC TREATMENT OF MENTAL ILLNESSES IN TEENAGERS

Unlike in allopathy, there is not just generalised treatment like tranquillisers, antidepressants irrespective of the specific cause.

In homeopathy, it is individualised and specific, especially in teenagers.

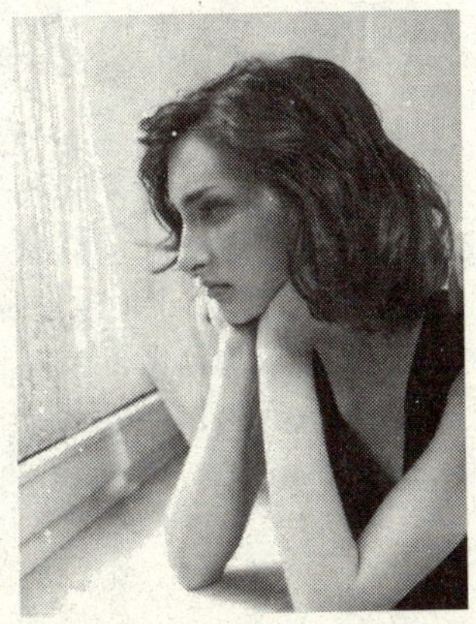

Mental Illness in Teenagers

My following paragraphs exclude treatment of Hyperactive Attention Deficit disorder, for which I had already dealt in my first book.

1. *Anger & Depression:*

This is the hallmark of emotional illnesses. Most of the crimes like suicides and homicides are committed during anger or depression, because during these emotions the rationality of mind is lost.

Very often it is the sexual frustration, or jilted in love affairs which lead to the above said negative emotions.

Ignatia and Aurum Met. are the king remedies in those who have lost interest in sex and every day's life activities. They do not want to mix with other people. These two remedies are for depression and sadness.

Staphysagaria and Acid phos. are particularly for anger due to sexual frustration in youngsters. If these are alternated with, Belladonna and Chamomilla, the results are magical.

Road rage amongst teenagers responds beautifully to the above four preparations.

2. *Insomnia (Loss of sleep):*

Kali phos and valleriana combination are excellent to give a sound sleep at night to these youngsters, without affecting their sexual desires unlike allopathic tranquillisers.

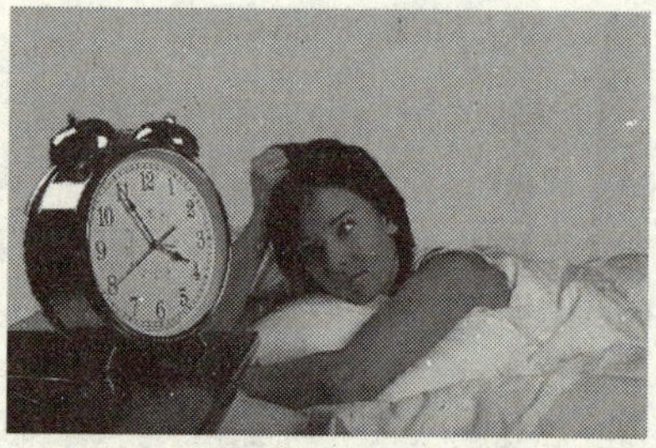

Loss of Sleep

3. *Hatred, Contempt, Jealousy, Apathy:*

These emotions are the worst enemy of mankind. These are often seen in jilted affairs, separation, divorces. Typical examples these days are amongst celebrities, like Britney Spears versus Kevin Federline, other of Paul McCartney versus Heather.

The most challenging cases which I had been asked to treat are those who have been in allopathic hands for years.

The most problematic cases are that of Schizophrenia and those who have been on Lithium preparations, the withdrawal of which cause serious aggravation.

Counselling:

It is an important adjuvant to homeopathic treatment, provided it is not given by the counsellor who himself is a mental patient.

In my experience, in India and abroad, majority of counsellors, psychologists and psychiatrists are patients themselves in the following way.

Psychologists: I was treating two young psychologists who were working in most reputed hospitals in Delhi– suffering themselves extreme degree of irritability, anger and depression.

Most of the psychiatrists who came for homeopathic treatment were themselves on tranquillisers and antidepressants.

As regards marriage counsellors, the less you ask the better it is. In the West, 80% of marriage counsellors themselves are divorcees.

Charity begins at home. Same applies with teachers. If they have to set example of controlled emotions, calmness, peacefulness, patience then they should be appointed to the job, not otherwise.

In the West, mere absence of their names in sex offenders or paedophillic registers, give them the visa for the job, without checking their personal and mental history.

My practical observations may be unpalatable, but it is imperative that employers should take note of these things if they have to control the present day hooliganism.

At the time of writing this subject, I read the news on Internet that a young boy shot 10 students in Finland. Last year, mass murder by a South Korean in USA is a livid example that there is something wrong with these theories of psychologists, drugs given by psychiatrists, somewhere there is a flaw.

Conclusively:

I will advise the policy of Stick and Carrot, as to how much to be given depends upon an individual's need. This type of handling and safe homeopathy are key anchor of my treatment.

◆◆◆

12.

EYE

DETACHMENT OF RETINA AND RETINA PIGMENTOSA

This condition is becoming common in epidemic proportions. The exact cause is not known but hereditary, high blood pressure is often attributed to be the causative factors.

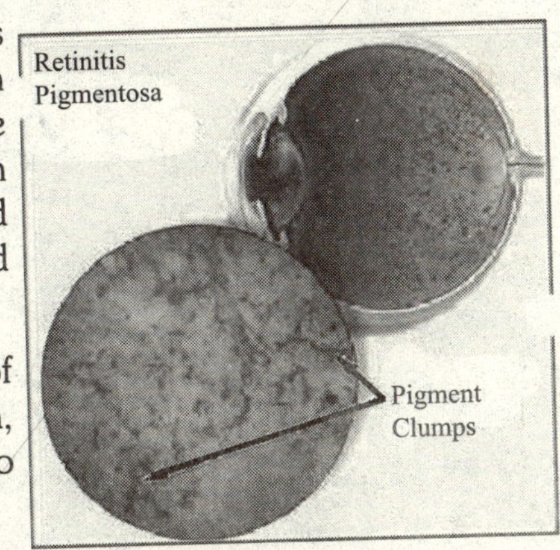

The dangerous site of its affection is the macula, which is very disabling to the patient.

Allopathy:

Laser treatment is considered to be a reasonably safe procedure, but this procedure has to be repeated often.

The procedure has its limitations as regards its cost and availability of facilities in India.

Both these things are out of bound for common man in India.

Homeopathy:

I have given the following combinations to many patients who had surgery, before or after repeated surgeries have failed.

A. Phosphorus is the head remedy and is of unquestionable value.

B. Combination of arnica+ and belladonna.

C. Combination of secale+hamammelis.

In macular degeneration, Carboneum sulphate is the drug of choice since this remedy is specific for special sensory nerve affinity.

CHALAZION

It is a very common condition of eyelid.

Allopathy:

The surgery in this case has a bad reputation because of its recurrence.

Pathologically, it is a retention cyst.

Case-1:

A 60-year-old man came to me if anything can be done as he had just been to topmost ophthalmologist who had suggested surgery and though it was a minor surgery, the risk was there since he was a diabetic and hypertensive. I asked him if he could bear with my homeo treatment for 2 months, he readily agreed.

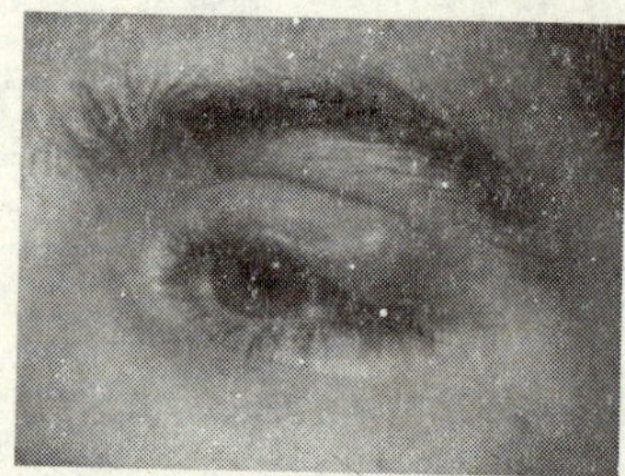

Eyelid

I commenced the treatment with Thuja 200 once a week followed by calcarea fluor. (hard) and acid nitric acid (jn.of skin and mucous membrane) in increasing potencies. In two months, the chalazion gradually disappeared.

CONJUNCTIVITIS

There are different types of conjunctivitis (bacterial, viral, allergic, infectious and traumatic) depending upon the causative factor.

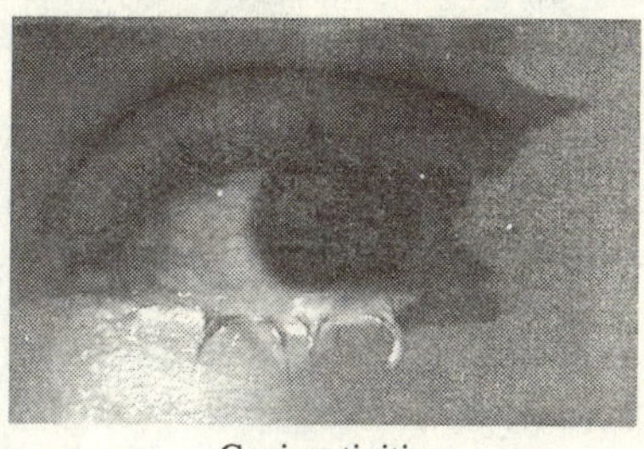

Conjunctivitis

Allopathy:

I have seen even in expert ophthalmologist's opinion, it is difficult to decide at a stage when the patient comes, unless there is obvious preceding history. As a result the ophthalmologist gives an eye drop which has all the ingredients (antibiotic, antihistaminic, anti-inflammatory).

But in allergic cases, the patient's eye reacts to the antibiotic making it more inflamed.

Such cases I have seen homeopathic given locally and internally is the safest approach.

Homeopathy:

Locally:

Euphrasia eye drops are of unquestionable value.

Internally:

Combination A. rhus tox + ruta + euphrasia

Combination B. arsenic alb + bell + apis

This combination has never failed whatever the causative factor is, except in heavily infective type of conjunctivitis or traumatic where the following combination does magic.

Combination C. arnica + symphytum:

The last combination I had to give as an emergency to my colleague's child in U.K. Though he took it reluctantly having no faith in homeopathy, he has no alternative since the child was allergic to host of other things.

DISEASES OF EYES

In the present edition, I will include diseases of eyes which are most formidable to treat and at the same time are beyond the reach of common man, financially or physical accessibility.

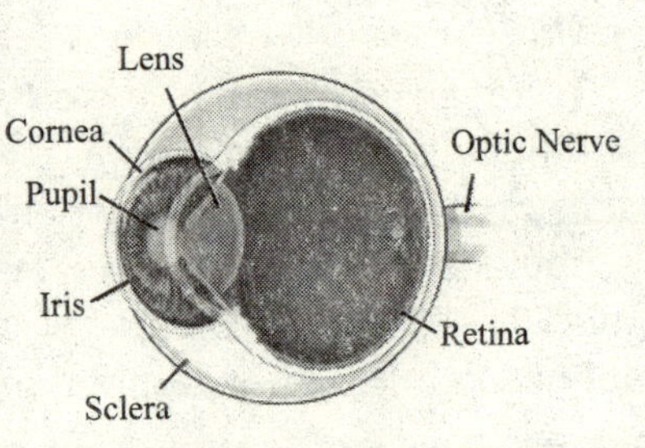

I had mentioned the common diseases like conjunctivitis and iridocyclitis.

In this chapter, I will mention the following:

1. Retinal detachment.
2. Retinal haemorrhage
3. Dry eyes
4. Glaucoma
5. Diplopia(double vision)—a part of multiple sclerosis
6. Optic nerve atrophy
7. Postcataract operation complications

RETINAL DETACHMENT AND RETINAL HAEMORRHAGE

The readers might scoff at the idea of homeopathic treatment for such diseases but when I was seeing these patients going again and again for laser treatments, I tried it.

In retinal detachment and haemorrhage, I give two groups of combinations in cyclic rotation.

A. arn.led.bell & hamm.

B. aur.mur and lach.

C. crotolas.h(in chronic recurrent he.)

I am surprised to see that despite the fact that retinal detachment is becoming very common, neither the cardiologist nor ophthalmologist realise, that in the dosage of aspirin prescribed by the cardiologist following angioplasty or coronary by-pass is one of the commonest causes of epidemic of retinal detachment. So the patient is between the devil and the deep sea.

In such cases, I feel 75 mg ecospirin is safer rather than 150 mg. At the same time, we counteract the side effect of aspirin with n.salicylate without antidoting its beneficial effect as a blood thinner.

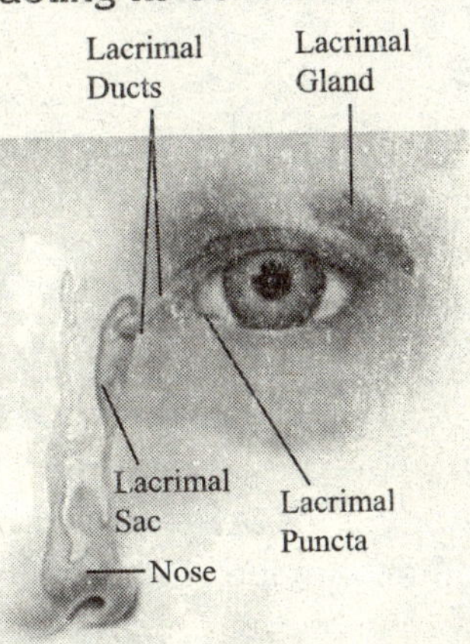

DRY EYES

This is one of the commonest complications after eye surgery, whether it is cataract or laser, since laser and post operative anti-inflammatory drugs and steroids take away the normal lubrication and the patient feels this complication as very annoying and he has to put eyedrops for life which is beyond the pocket of an ordinary person.

RETINITIS PIGMENTOSA, THROMBOSIS, DENERATION

I have treated innumerable cases provided they come early rather than after repeated laser treatments with adhesions and scarring.

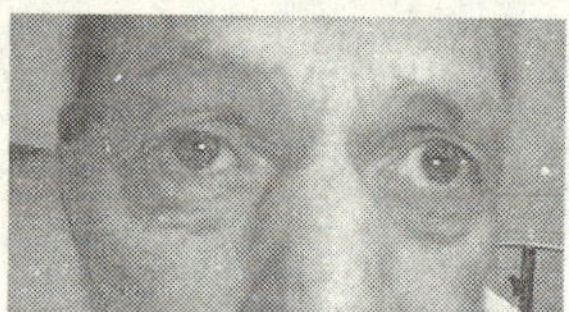

Retinitis Pigmentosa

Homeopathy:

Phosphorus, Hamm. and nux vomica are of immense benefit and give excellent results.

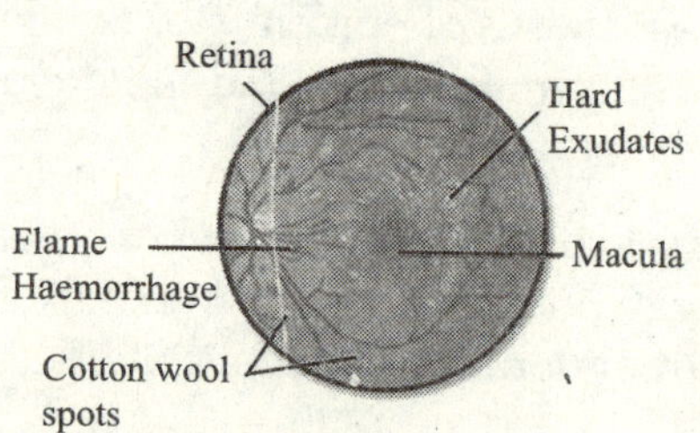

HYPERTENSIVE AND DIABETIC RETINOPATHY

It is imperative to treat the underlying cause in both these conditions before giving homeopathy for these complications.

Homeopathy: Apis, lach, glono and bell.

DIPLOPIA (DOUBLE VISION)

This symptom could be very benign or a symptom of serious underlying deep-seated disease. After having dealt with quite a few cases, having excluded underlying tumour of brain or

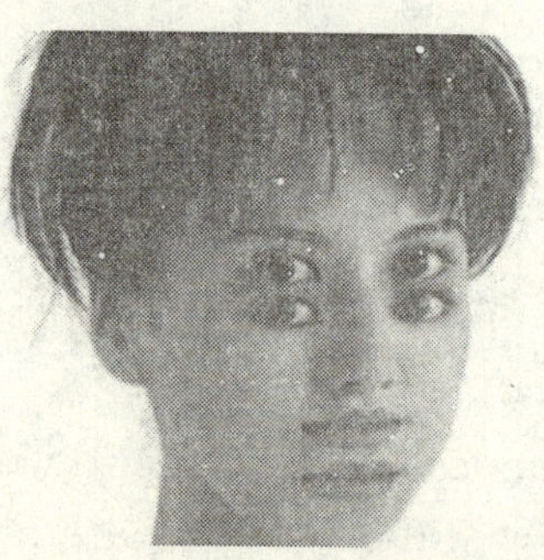

Diplopia (Double Vision)

post-meningitis complication by ophthalmologists as the cause, I have taken up such cases.

Very often, it is one of the symptom complex of multiple sclerosis for which these patients have been made a mess by treatment with repeated courses of steroids in reputed hospitals in Delhi and abroad.

The treatment of multiple sclerosis has been dealt under a separate heading in this book.

However, since phosphorus is the head remedy, one must exclude T.B. before treating with phosphorus since this is contraindicated in T.B.

SUBSTITUTE TO POSTOPERATIVE ALLOPATHIC DRUGS AFTER EYE SURGERY

Since most of the drugs used postoperatively are NSAID preparations which cause allergic reactions and to counteract allergic reactions whether skin or asthma, they give cetrizine and steroids, and to counteract the acidity caused by NSAID preparations or steroids, they give antacids like pantoprazole or acid which again cause dryness.

So the extreme dryness is caused by:

A. Drugs given for inflammation caused by surgery.

B. Drugs given to counteract the side effects of these anti-inflammatory or painkillers.

C. Laser for retinal surgery: the heat created by its use (despite the counter measures included in the laser machine).

It pains me to learn that even the educated class of people do not ask the ophthalmologists, nor the ophthalmologists explain to the patient beforehand that there will be lifelong dryness following surgery.

AUTHOR'S REGIME OF PRE AND POST–OPERATIVE HOMEO-REMEDIES IN EYE OPERATIONS

Pre: Combination of arnica, calendula and hypericum and rhus tox.

Post: Combination of aconite bryonia and ignatia for pain in head and temples.

Senega for absorption of lens debris.

Strontium for objects appearing tinged with blood.

OPTIC NERVE ATROPHY

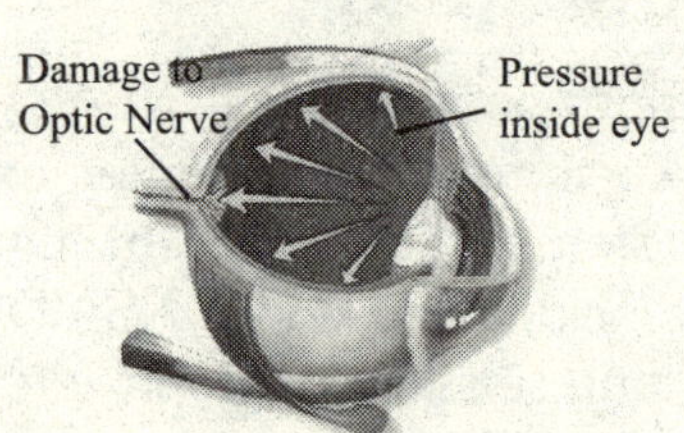

In the experience of the author, there is no treatment in allopathy for this condition.

Homeopathy:

In my experience, Carboneum sulphate is of unquestionable value provided the patient comes early.

GLAUCOMA AND OPTIC NERVE ATROPHY

Although there are so many advances in the treatment of glaucoma (black cataract) in allopathy, still lots of cases proceed to malignant variety eventually leading to blindness.

The following is an interesting case I was confronted with for the first time and was very happy to get good results as there was hardly any hope after seven years treatment with allopathy and after having spent lakhs of rupees in retinal MRI and retinal angiography repeatedly, when in their hearts the ophthalmologists knew that they cannot do anything.

Case:

A young man of 37 years of age had a severe car accident 10 years ago, following which he developed severe glaucoma and optic nerve atrophy.

The top private eye institute's glaucoma specialist was giving the usual anti-glaucoma eye drops and of course, he had nothing to offer for optic nerve atrophy.

Homeopathy:

1. Arnica 1M to start the treatment followed by: (Head injury)
2. Phosphorus
3. Gelsemium
4. Agaricus
5. Nat. sulph(head injury complication)
6. Carboneum sulph (cranial nerve)

Beyond my expectations, the patient had improvement in vision in 2 weeks. However, the treatment is being continued with antidotes to allopathic medicines which had already been given.

◆◆◆

13.

INJURIES (MODEL CURE)

The history of this young man involved in a severe car accident while on an official trip to Delhi from Singapore is a livid example to prove that both allopathy and homeopathy have their respective roles in certain situations, while indispensable and complementary to each other in other situations.

Allopathy:

Case-1:

This young handsome boy had a compound fracture of ankle, laceration of upper eyelid involving the eyebrow. It was a ghastly scene.

ANKLE

Open reduction and plating was done for the ankle injury. According to the orthopaedic surgeon, after finishing the operation chances of healing and complete recovery were bleak since talus was involved which has no blood supply of its own.

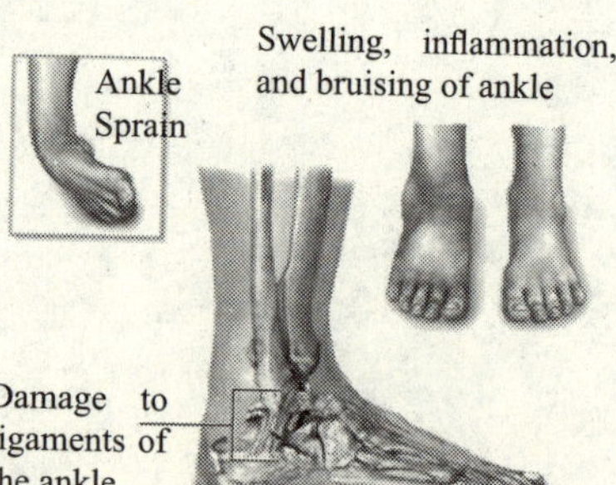

Apart from plaster and antibiotics and anti-inflammatory drugs, it was left to nature.

Homeopathy:

Based on my knowledge of anatomy, physiology and pathology, I gave the following two groups of homeo combinations:

A. Rhus tox, ruta, arnica, ledum pal, calendula and hypericum.

Reason:

For muscles (rhus tox), ligaments (ruta), pressure on nerves (hypericum), open injury more susceptible to infection (calendula) ledum pal to prevent tetanus and long-term residual local oedema.

B: *For bony union:* I gave combination of symphytum and calcarea phos

The orthopaedic surgeon was amazed to see the check X-ray after removing the plaster and plates.

EYE INJURY

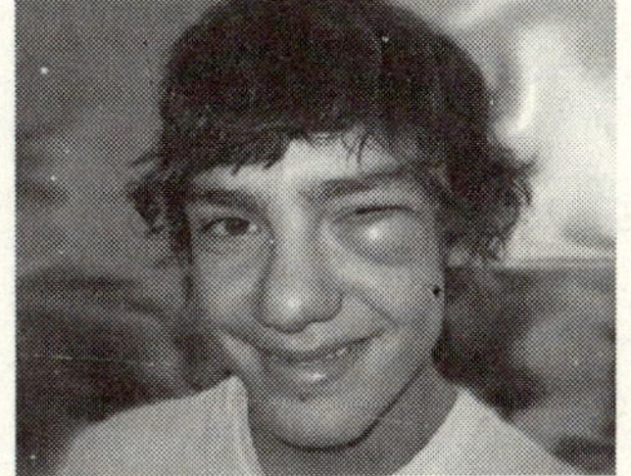

After the eye surgery was performed by ophthalmologist plastic surgeon and general ophthalmic surgeon jointly, the patient recovered but two unsightly complications developed.

A. Ectropian at certain places and entropian at other places.

B. Cicatrices at other situations and keloid at other places, he being fair complexion.

Here the ophthalmologic plastic surgeon and general plastic surgeon were unable to promise any better results by further surgery.

Homeopathy:

Here I gave graphites, calcarea fluor, causticum in different potencies.

Despite all these major surgical operations, the best results could only be achieved because of strong belief of this gentleman in homeopathy and positive thinking.

After having achieved the best cosmetic and functional results, he got a beautiful wife and is happily settled in Singapore.

◆◆◆

14.

AUTO-IMMUNE DISEASES

This label has become very popular amongst specialists and super-specialists. So to say, these specialists and immunologists have labelled the following disease as autoimmune.

Firstly as an allopath and as ENT surgeon, having dealt with allergic conditions of nose and chest in Western countries for more than thirty years, with all the desensitisation vaccines, from Beecham Bencard, I have arrived at the conclusion that homeopathic dilutions if properly selected are far better, safer, cheaper and more convenient than desensitisation by allopathic means.

The autoimmune diseases labelled by chest specialists, dermatologists, gastroenterologists, endocrinologists and rheumatologists are as below:

1. Allergic rhinitis
2. Bronchial asthma
3. Ulcerative colitis
4. Eczema
5. Rheumatoid arthritis
6. Thyroid(hypothyroidism)

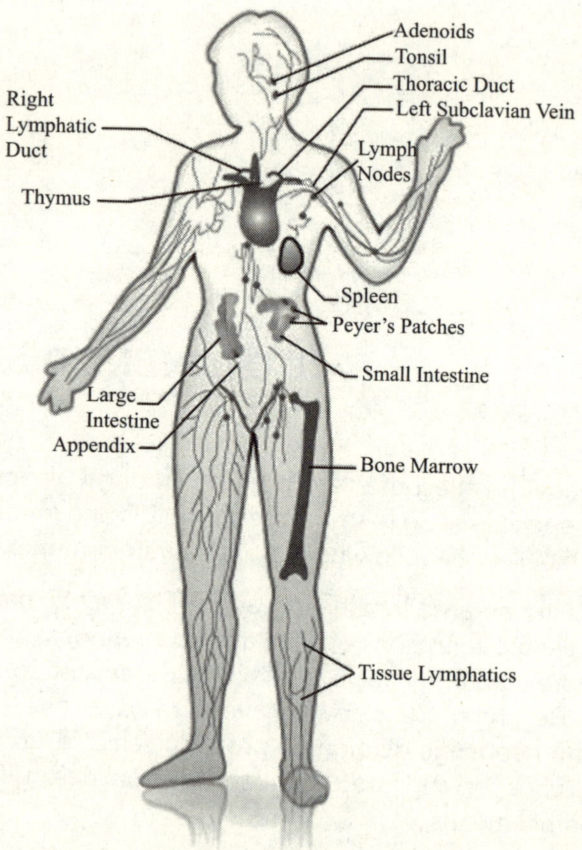

Immune System

Aetiology: Most of these cases, to their surprise, it maybe, in my experience is caused by allopathic vaccines and drugs since I have counteracted and treated them–with success– on the basis of this aetiology.

Mechanism of causation by Allopaths:

1. Infantile eczema or atopic dermatitis is caused by these vaccination–whether it is the base of vaccine or other extraneous factors in vaccine, I have dealt in the last edition of my book.

2. Allopathic drugs, especially, brufen, advil and other NSAID preparations except nimulid.

These often lead to asthma or dermatitis(eczema, erythema nodosum etc).

Various antibiotics are notorious for causing allergic reaction.

Allopathic treatment of autoimmune is the worst treatment and eventually leads to end of no return.

The only treatment with these super-specialists is antiallergics, cetrizine, avil, piriton, allegra claritin, nukast and if no relief then steroids, whether orally or in depot form (medrone in UK and medrol in India). These patients become their permanent customers. Suppressing reactions (which are caused by allopathic treatment), in my experience has lead to rheumatoid arthritis, sciatica, paralysis, multiple sclerosis.

Patients have come to me, for homeopathy, after having treatment from all these super-specialists with allopathy and by homeopaths who base their treatment only on symptoms rather than complete approach (examination and diagnostic tools as well).

Such allopathic treatment certainly make the treatment with homeopathy more difficult than those who had no allopathic treatment.

I would like to request the public at large that before they start allopathic treatment such as steroids or methotrexate for arthritis, they should ask the doctor as to whether the diseases created by these drugs are not worse than the diseases for which these drugs are being given.

I had innumerable patients with side effects of methotrexate with permanent fibrosis of lungs and then being referred to pulmonologists, again he simply puts them on heavy doses of steroids.

The author has reserved steroid only in case of anaphylactic shock or some operative complication needing steroid. Sometimes severe urticaria needs steroid, but then soon after lifesaving steroid dose, they should go on homeopathy treatment.

◆◆◆

15.

COSMETIC (PLASTIC MEDICINE)

The value of this greatest asset of a woman can be appreciated if the readers refer to page 103 of my book 'Homeopathy Cures Where Allopathy Fails'.

Under its heading following conditions are enlisted:

Breasts

Small atrophic

Pendulous especially after breastfeeding

Very large heavy breast

Large belly especially after delivery

Allopathic Treatment:

Plastic surgery despite being very advanced, still thousands of cases are in the court against plastic surgeons and silicon manufacturing companies.

One should not undermine the immediate or late complications of plastic surgery.

Infection, scarring, deep scar, asymmetrical breasts, burst silicon implant, the tremendous cost of operation.

Homeopathy:

In my experience, each case needs specific remedy and a particular potency.

Atrophic Breast:

Case-1:

18-year-old girl is emaciated and skinny with enlarged cervical glands, I gave iodum 30 and that worked wonders for her.

Case-2:

42-year-old woman, very irritable, unmarried depressed, conscious of her 30 size wanted to marry but was too conscious of the small size of her breasts. She was extremely irritable.

I gave staphysagaria 200 which not only increased her breast but also changed her temperament.

Case-3:

18-year-old chloreatic girl, highly strung, hypochondriac and hysterical with atrophic breast was given ignatia and aurum met, she was a different girl in six-month-time.

Case-4:

Small breast, large shoulders and large buttocks, stunning beauty.

I gave calcarea carb for six months in changing potency and she was different girl in six-month-time.

Case-5:

In many young women with penduious breasts after delivery, mercurious vivax and pulsatilla have made a tremendous difference in the appearance and firmness of their breasts.

Very Large Breasts:

Case-6:

40-year-old gynae-obstetrician came complaining that her very large breasts are troublesome while she is operating on patients.

I gave Nux Vomica in different potencies, at increasing intervals, and she attained size 38 and got confidence in herself.

Case-7:

Obesity with Large belly:

Calcarea carb and nux vomica in different constitutions have brought normality in their appearance.

◆◆◆

16.

WOMEN DISEASES

OBESITY, THYROID DYSFUNCTION AT MENOPAUSE

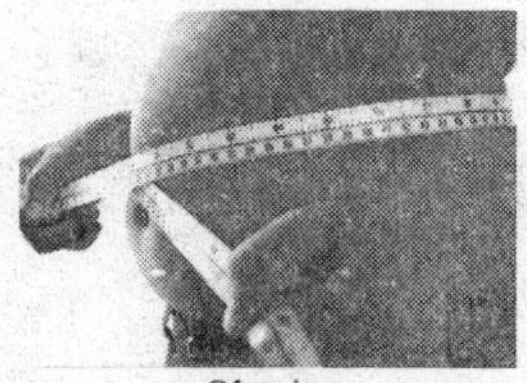
Obesity

The above two ailments have gained epidemic proportions and I have observed that gynae-obstetricians, endocrinologists and physicians label it due to hormonal disturbances and overeating.

1. Overeating and lack of exercise may be true in 10% of cases.

2. Stiffness of joints and rheumatism force certain women to lack of exercise, thus leading to increase in weight.

3. The most disturbing thing is that hypothyroidism cases are coming in epidemic proportions and are coming at much younger age than what they used to be.

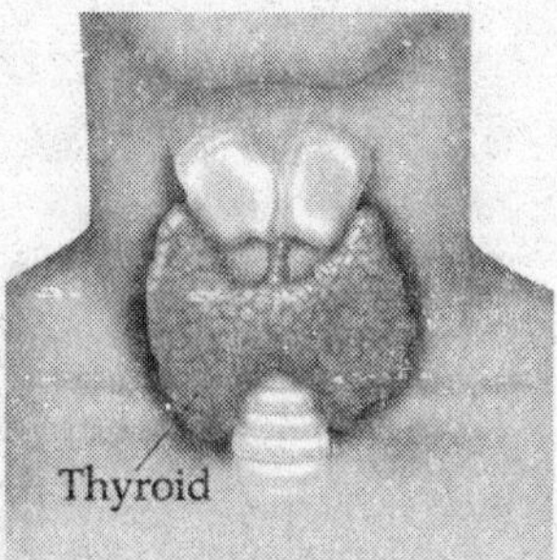
Thyroid

4. In my informal talk with the above specialists on the reason of increasing number

of hypothyroidism, they do not agree with my following observations.

Allopathy:

Aetiology:

In my experience, advances in various modern hormonal preparations and allopathic drugs, stresses and strain of life lead to Thyroid Dysfunction.

Hormones given for irregular periods.

Hormones given for sterility.

Contraceptive pills.

All these preparations interfere with thyroid and ovarian glands.

Stresses and strain interfere with these glandular functions by excessive stimulation of hypothalamus —Anterior Pituitary— excessive stimulation of thyroid and ovary.

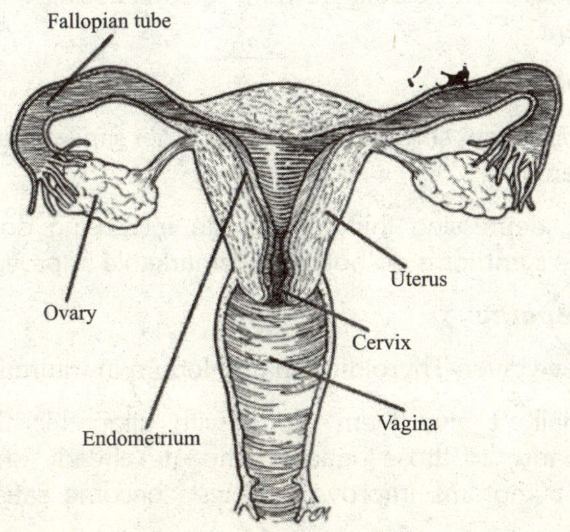

Polycystic ovaries are the gifts given by these enthusiastic allopaths prescribing hormonal preparations at the stroke of hammer, maybe steroids, oestrogen-progesterone.

I would like to emphasise the point that it is often the rule rather than exception that thyroid tests do not come positive at least for 3-4 years since the onset of sub clinical Myxoedema.

The early symptoms of hypothyroidism are:

- Increase in weight
- Depression
- Irritability
- Disturbed sleep
- Lethargy and weakness
- Skin rashes

Investigations:

Blood test, ultrasound, ECG and isotope studies where indicated, should be done before deciding on line of treatment.

Allopathy:

Thyronorm, eltroxin and various other similar preparations are given.

The depressing thing is despite increasing dosage, the patient's symptoms do not show remarkable improvement.

Homeopathy:

I have given Thyroidinium and Iodum in trituration.

Initially I give them along with allopathic thyronorm particularly to those patients who are already on it. Then as the symptoms improve and tests become satisfactory, I taper allopathy and eventually stop thyronorm but continue homeopathic remedies.

Frigidity in Women and Impotency in Men.

These are the common causes of marital discord especially at climatic age, leading to separation and divorces.

Frigidity in Women: Impotency in Men:

Amongst Indian women, religious fanaticism is the common cause of frigidity.

The wrong teachings by so-called self appointed moral messengers of God are the causative factors in majority of cases.

Allopathy:

Present view is that Viagra also works in women by increasing the blood supply to their genital areas.

But everybody is aware of the side effects, especially in those having angina, low blood pressure or hot flushes.

The other common side effect of Viagra is haemorrhoids (piles).

Homeopathy:

Lycopodium in high potency and onosmodium are of unquestionable value, to enhance the sexual desire and arousal in both the sexes. The trick of the magic lies in the potency in a particular individual.

◆◆◆

17.

MISCELLANEOUS DISEASES

PAROTID GLAND FISTULA WITH CALCULUS

Model Cure:

This is an unusual case of an NRI young girl who came from abroad and was having discharge from parotid duct, spilling on the cheek more so while eating food. Ultra sound of parotid gland revealed a calculus. So I was to treat this girl's calculus and fistula of 2 years duration.

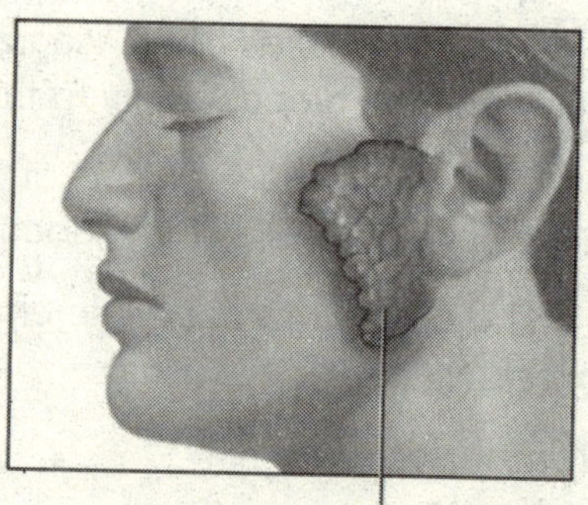

Swollen parotid gland

The father refused the operation abroad despite having all the facilities, since no surgeon could give guarantee regarding the safety of facial nerve during operation.

Homeopathy:

I treated this case effectively utilising my ENT experience in allopathy and homeopathy. I gave the following combinations:

A. Acid nitric because of type of discharge.

B. Because of fibrosis of parotid duct, I gave cal. fluor, causticum and clematis (for stricture of the duct)

C. Belladonna and Calendula – for inflammation and infection respectively.

I am sure many of homeopath colleagues would have suggested silicea–the standard treatment, but I did not like expulsion on the face and permanent scarring.

It took six months when the patient was 80% recovered at the time of submitting this case for publication.

HOMEOPATHY IN CORONARY ARTERY DISEASE

In this life-threatening ailment, I have seen even the protagonists of homeopathy are reluctant to take and they give preference usually to allopathy.

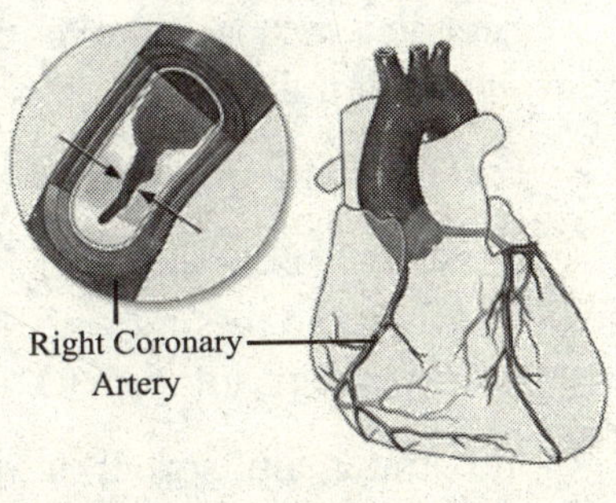

The most important point to remember is not every case is the same with this diagnosis.

Secondly, allopathic diagnostic tools are a must and an individual's emotional set up, the degree of underlying pathology are the deciding factors.

I personally am of the opinion to give first choice to surgical treatment (angioplasty or coronary bypass), if one has to lead quality of life, provided the surgery is done by honest, competent interventional cardiologist or cardiac surgeon. I am dealing in the present chapter of those who get recurrent blockage after bypass or angioplasty.

They get demoralised and do not want to undergo the repeat procedure. I have patients coming to me after recurrence of the disease, after having had the surgery by top cardiac surgeons abroad or here.

My following homeopathic treatment is for recurrent cases:

1. CrategusQ and arjuna.t-Q 5 drops of each 3 times daily after meals, for a long time.

Reason: It keeps the arteries clear of clogging. It regulates the heart rate.

In comparison, allopathic treatment by cardiologists like beta blockers give various swings such as:

Feeling weak, low, fluctuation in blood pressure and pulse, despite what they claim it is protective to heart.

2. Essentia aura gold drops twice daily.

Reason: It is really gold for the heart. It controls stress, clotting, blood pressure and heart rate. Cactus ingredient is very good antispasmodic.

In comparison, sorbitrate does not suit all patient because of its lowering of blood pressure and severe headache in some cases. It can cause postural hypotension which itself can lead to clotting.

3. Arnica and spigelia once daily before going for a walk.

Reason: It is par excellence in preventing clotting, antispasmodic for coronary arteries, dissolves the clots if any.

4. Five phos 3 times daily

Reason: It is a tranquilliser, antispasmodic, brain and heart tonic.

In comparison, tranquillisers like alprax, alzolam, ativan, play hell with elderly people, apart from affecting alertness leading to drowsiness and habit forming.

Adverse effects are visible due to medication of post angioplasty and coronary bypass surgery.

The common medicines prescribed which are indispensable are:

Ecospirin (in one or other form)and clopidogril (deplatt): These preparations are meant to keep the blood thin, so that the blood keeps flowing in the coronary arteries without any danger of clotting:

Following are the adverse effects of ecospirin and clopiodogril:

1. *Bleeding:* The bleeding can be from any outlet of the body: it can be from nose, per rectum, urine or haematemesis.

   Any small cut or injury can cause excessive bleeding.

   A.C.T (Author's Comments and Treatment):

As an ENT surgeon, I have seen hundreds of patients coming with epistaxis (bleeding from nose), bleeding from ear, deep to Tympanic membrane leading to sudden deafness.

The bleeding due to blood thinners from any site (urine, per rectum, retinal or intracranial) however, more often than not, these do not come to the notice of the interventional cardiologist or cardiac surgeon. The patients usually go to the specific specialists and many times such bleeding proves fatal as blood transfusions are not without risks.

Allopathy:

The only treatment is to stop aspirin and clopidogrel: It takes about three days before the effect of aspirin wears off.

But the problem is we will have to restart aspirin and clopidogrel after a few days, since heart and brain health has a priority over other things.

To give blood transfusion in such cases is not without risks as it involves elderly people with poor cardiac and renal function.

Homeopathy:

There are many preparations mentioned but author has found hammemelis and carboveg to be effective.

My colleague Dr. Kulbhushan Bharadwaj with his extensive experience has found ipecacque to be more effective.

The author is on research to find a homeopathic blood thinner which should take the place of aspirin and clopidogrel.

2. Tinnitus (noises in ears, nerve deafness):

The author sees hundreds of such patients in ENT outpatients in U.K. 50% of cases per clinic are of Meniere's syndrome (above symptoms). This is due to aspirin.

Allopathy:

Absolute failure in the experience of author, Tinnitus masker as the treatment is worse than the disease.

Tranquillisers are simply a smokescreen against fire and do not treat the cause and incapacitate him for work, since it leads to lethargy and drowsiness.

Homeopathy:

The author has given his treatment guidelines based on his combination of knowledge and experience as an ENT surgeon and Homeopathy:

Natrum salicylate – I have found natrum salicylate is very specific to counteract side effects of aspirin and not the beneficial effect of aspirin as a thinner.

ADVERSE EFFECTS OF ANTI-TUBERCULAR REGIME

This is an interesting case in that it depicts how the super-speciality of allopathy causes diseases rather than curing.

Case:

A young man of 35 years was diagnosed with Potts disease (T.B. of spine) at D-12 and L1.

He was put on ATT and after two months of treatment he had no relief in the spine, but he got in addition dangerous side-effects of the ATT drugs as follows:

1. His kidney failed.
2. Due to Ethambutol, he got partial blindness of left eye and optic nerve atrophy. All the retinal investigations done by ophthalmologists gave no assurance and gave bad prognosis.

To make things worse, super-specialist neurologist of a reputed private hospital in Delhi put him on aspirin to keep the blood thin after the surgery on the spine failed.

As a result, he got after 6 weeks treatment after which he developed brain haemorrhage resulting in hemiplegia.

Now I had to treat him following allopathic induced diseases by so-called super-specialists of top institutions who report only successful cases but not the various incurable diseases caused by them.

Homeopathy:

A. *Kidney Failure:* With 132 blood urea and 7 mg creatinine, I gave cuprum arsneicum, elserum and terebinth.

However, as additional help, I gave diuretic (R-58) for oedema and puffiness of whole body.

B. *Eye:* For optic nerve atrophy, I gave carboneum sulphate and for retinal haemorrhage, I gave phosphorus and hammemelis, after the patient failed to respond to laser.

C. *Paralysis of Lower legs:* I gave plumbum and lathyrus

D. *Neuritis and Neuralgia of legs due to pressure on spinal nerves:* I gave combination of cimcifuga, hypericum and oxalic acid.

E. Stiffness and rigidity of all the limbs: My combination of cal.fl. caust. and thiosin. removed stiffness by 30%.

HOMEO-REMEDIES FOR OLD AGE DISEASES

1. *Loss of memory:* Baryta carb, Ambra and Anacardium are of unquestionable value.
2. *Prostatic hypertrophy:* Conium, Baryta carb and Sabal serrulata have never failed.
3. *To rejuvenate skin and joints:* Thiosinamun in different potencies is of great help.
4. *In Cataract:* Calcarea flo. and Thios delays the onset of cataract.

DISEASES CAUSED BY COMMONLY USED ALLOPATHIC DRUGS

1. Painkillers like brufen, ibuprofen, advil, mefal, voveran, diclofenac and methotrexate, if taken frequently as usually the case is leads to kidney damage. That is the reason, these days kidney failure cases are coming at younger age.

   I wish the doctors warn the patients or the patients should ask the doctors the side effects of these drugs.

2. Skin eczema, in its worst form, is caused by the above painkillers.

These cases become more complicated by the use of steroid creams and ointments by allopaths, leading to suppression, making the fertile ground for eczema.

3. Rheumatoid arthritis.
4. Gastric Ulcer and Colitis are the other complications caused by these drugs.
5. Superspecialists-Rheumatologists: These rheumatologists relieve the pain at the expense of causing fibrosis of lungs, liver damage, severe pigmentation of the skin. This is the stage when the patients have come to me for homeopathic treatment. Most of these side-effects are caused by methotrexate – a very favourite drug with immunologists and rheumatologists.

A.C.T.(Author's Comments & Treatment):

In my experience, most of autoimmune diseases are caused by allopathic treatment with suppressant drugs (painkillers, antiallergic and steroids).

Prolonged use of these drugs lead to even bone marrow depression.

Homeopathy:

The treatment has been mentioned of such complications in the previous paragraphs.

Some more diseases caused by commonly used allopathic drugs:

1. Antacids (omenaprazole, ocid, pantoprazole): Commonly used for oesophagitis and acid reflux are taken rountinely by the patients for long periods without realising their side effects. These are also given to those with diagnosis of helicobacter pylori. The side effects are arthralgia, myalgia, skin reactions and dry mouth.

2. Lomotil (Loperamide): This used to be a very popular drug in the West. Now, when they have banned, doctors are still using it in India. The most dangerous side effect of it is paralytic Ileus (paralysis of intestine).

3. Salazine (Aminosalycilate): Commonly used in I.B.S. (Irritable Bowel Syndrome) and ulcerative colitis. I have seen patients on this drug coming to me with blood disorder like purpura haemorrhagicaca (bleeding in any part of eye, conjuctiva, retina).

4. Antidepressants: The following common side effects must be kept in mind, before starting these addictive drugs.

a. Obesity

b. Constipation

c. Reduces the libido in both the sexes

d. Parkinsonism

e. Dystopia and Dyskinesia: Abnormal face and bodily movements. Involuntary movements of face and tongue.

f. Drowsiness, agitation, excitement, insomnia, dry mouth, constipation.

g. Endocrine side-effects: Menstrual disturbances. Gynaecoastia (enlargement of breast in males) atrophy of breast in female.

h. Blood Dyscrasia

i. Eye changes: Corneal lense opacity, purple pigmentation of cornea and retina.

DISEASES CAUSED BY ALLOPATHS THROUGH UNNECESSARY PHOBIAS ABOUT HEART AND CANCER

It is absolutely correct to have a health and blood check up from reliable, honest physician and a laboratory of repute.

May I point out the fallacies of the present day dangers of unnecessary phobias created by so-called neurotic physicians and greedy laboratories, leading to the following diseases:

1. Cardiac neurosis is one of the common ailment created by the present day physicians. I have seen some neurotic physicians will bring any symptom of the body, maybe nail or stomach that 'may not be due to heart' and all the unnecessary investigations.
2. The other example is headache, instead of thinking about the commonest cause like sinus, error of refraction or tension. Headache will straight away go to MRI, CT scan, focusing the patient's attention, as if something is serious. This leads to anxiety neurosis.
3. After causing anxiety neurosis in an apparently healthy person, he will be referred to a psychiatrist. Then God save the patients from those addictive drugs.
4. Gynae-obs, once were very enthusiastic about removing the ovaries, even looking apparently and hormonal disturbances, thus putting them on HRT, which has its own dangers of causing cancer of breast and strokes. I am pleased they are realising it now but still top gynae are still causing ablation of ovaries which are apparently healthy.
5. Finally, do not consider doctors as the last word, I have seen hundreds of cases with wrong biopsy and blood

report has undergone wrong treatment. Even the other day, it was in the press that AIIMS has to pay Rs. 5 lakh for removing a healthy breast because the biopsy report given was wrong.

6. A week ago, I had a case who was taken to Sloan kettering hospital in New York, after she had been operated upon in a reputed hospital in Delhi and here the pathologist reported benign, while kettering confirmed it is the fourth stage malignant.

7. Similarly, a young lady due to injury (not severe) to spine was brought to Delhi, the neurosurgeon operated on her which lead to paralysis. While the report was malignant at the hospital where she was operated upon, it turned out to benign at Tata in Mumbai. However, the lady suffered permanent paralysis due to operation.

There is endless list of such diseases caused by doctors.

DISEASES CAUSED BY HOMEOPATHS AND HOMEOPATHIC REMEDIES

It will not be out of place to warn the public that everything is not safe as they presume or no side effects as commonly thought.

Homeopathy in good hands is a boon.

If it is used with caution and safely with experience, it can work wonders. I will say in the same breath that I have seen unqualified but experienced homeopaths have done wonders which sometimes the qualified could not do.

It is a pity that sometimes a clear surgical condition is being treated by homeopaths of repute, for years, thinking it not advisable to send to a surgeon, spoiling the case.

As an example, deviated nasal septum of the nose or a big perforation in Tympanic membrane needs surgery. Like that there are innumerable examples.

The same way I have seen proving and diseases caused by repeated doses of very high potency of antipsoric or antipsychotic remedies.

HOMEOPATHY AND ALLOPATHY —FRIENDS OR FOES

I have seen these two pathies have confused both the allopaths and homeopaths. My advice on the following lines will help both sides of physicians.

It is a common experience, many patients who have been taking allopathy for months and years, when not getting response try to seek help from homeopaths.

Without realising the implication of their decision, some will ask to continue allopathy as well. Others will straight away stop the allopathy, without realising the action of those allopathic drugs. It is also true vice-versa, when some allopaths will stop homeopathy, taking it as a placebo or just small pills are of no significance, while others will say to continue homeopathy as well knowing intuitively that their allopathy is also of not much benefit.

To solve this problem, physician must know the antidotal and complementary effect of both homeopathic remedies and allopathic remedies.

To go into details of this is not within the scope of this book, however, I will mention just a few important ones so that physicians should be on the guard.

1. Steroids and Betablockers should not be stopped suddenly.
2. Antiallergics in allopathy like cetrizine, allegra, avil, actifed, dcold and steroids should never be given with

homeo remedies used for allergy such as arsenic alb, natrum mur, phosphorus.

3. Brochodilators like asthaline, ventolin, deriphylline, theophylline should not be used with ipecacque, mag. Phos, colocynth, blatta-Q.
4. Painkillers like brufen, advin, meftal, combiflam, proxyvon should not be used with along with homeo: medicines like belladonna, bryonnia, mag. Phos.
5. Hepar sulph and silicea should not be used along with antibiotics. They are contradictory in their effects.

DEPRESSION DUE TO SEXUAL MISCONCEPTIONS IN MARRIED COUPLES

Various misconceptions about the duration of sexual intercourse has led to many men and women going into depression, leading to impotency and sexual frustration among women.

The research has been done in this aspect in Australia and I quote from that study, which will help to remove the myths and truth about sex.

It has been agreed that the best sexual intercourse lasts between 7 to 13 minutes.

According to Eric Corty from Pennsylvania, three minutes sex is adequate.

The ideal length of time to have penetrating sex, with random samples from Americans and Canadians, is 7 to 13 minutes.

The purpose of reproducing this study in my book is to calm many couples coming to me asking for homeopathic aphrodisiacs rather than allopathic owing to the side effects of allopathic drugs.

This will calm down many couples who have unrealistic beliefs that healthy sex should last long.

'In the fantasy model of male sexuality, men have large penises, rock-hard erections and can sustain sexual activity all night long,' says Corty in News.com.au.

It appears many men and women hold this fantasy.

The result from the present study by providing a realistic, not a fantasy model of sexuality, is useful in treating people with sexual concerns and dysfunction, thus preventing the onset of sexual dysfunction. The above study has been published in the International Journal of Sexual Medicine.

Homeopathy:

The author has found very satisfying results in such couples after counselling and giving Acid Phos and Onosmodium in high potencies.

SURGERY AND HOMEOPATHY —FRIENDS, NOT ENEMIES

As I have mentioned in the preface of the book that homeopathy can be complementary and not antisurgery as I will explain in a few examples out of many cases where I routinely apply.

I categorically differ from orthodox view that either medicines (homeopathy or allopathy)or surgery.

The author uses homeopathy as a routine before and after ENT surgery, thereby reducing the need of allopathic medicines, thereby less side-effects and morbidity in a patient.

The homeo remedies used depend upon the type of surgery I do.

1. Cases involving cartilage and bone such as deviated nasal septum–Ruta and rhus tox is a must in addition to arnica.

2. In fracture of nose, after setting by surgical manoeuvre, Calc.phos and symphytum is a boon.
3. In mastoid surgery, for chronic ear infection, calendula in high potency following surgery is a must, to prevent any intracranial complication, like meningitis.
4. In soft tissue injury repair like lip or face,before and after repair, ledum pal, hypericum, rhus tox and calendula are of unquestionable value.

OSTEOPOROSIS

This word has become very familiar, especially in women owing to postmenopausal bone density loss due to calcium depletion.

Diagnostic Radialogists are having a heyday by getting every woman to get bone density and then labelling as Osteoporosis and putting them on calcium (Gem cai and other such fascinating names).

I feel nothing like having natural calcium rather than these pharmacological calcium which may not get absorbed or assimilated properly, or may form kidney stones.

Now the doctors have come up with novel preparation which is not hormonal in chemistry.

A.C.T. (Author's Comments and Treatment):

Bisphosphonates: It had become very popular for a few years in the West until recently when its side effects (proved) started showing up, then it has been dumped in India.

1. Cancer of oesophagus (windpipe) is one of the dangerous side effect by its use.
2. It has been found it increases the quantity of bone and not the quality of bone, thus fractures can still occur.

DEEP VENOUS THROMBOSIS (D.V.T.)

Here there is clotting (thrombosis) of blood in deep veins of the calf muscles.

This condition is becoming common even in younger people owing to stagnation of blood in leg veins, and prolonged operations. Although precautions are taken to prevent clotting by calf massagers.

The prolong flights are also responsible for D.V.T. if the legs are not moved for long periods.

Allopathy:

Anticoagulants are the mainstay treatment, but this treatment has its own dangers of excessive bleeding.

This treatment also requires repeated blood tests for prothrombin, b.t and ct.

The biggest bugbear of D.V.T. is pulmonary embolism which can cause instantaneous death.

Homeopathy:

I find arnica, lachesis and bothrops of unquestionable value, with no side effects.

◆◆◆

18.

MODERN CONCEPTS

REMOVAL OF OVARIES, OESTROGENS AND DEMENTIA

Recent findings of Dr. Walter Rocca of the Mayo Clinic in Maryland have given a blow to the enthusiastic Gynae-Obs, who often believe in removal of ovaries while doing hysterectomies.

According to Dr. Rocca, removal of ovaries before menopause almost doubles the risk of developing dementia in old age.

According to her, oestrogens protect the brains of younger women.

ATTENTION DEFICIENT HYPERACTIVE DISORDER (ADHD)

Here is another U-turn in the so-called scientifically proved drugs.

According to health reporter of Times (U.K.), Ritalin commonly prescribed drug for the above disorder has caused heavy financial strain on the health expenditure despite its serious side effects like depression, drowsiness, epilepsy and high blood pressure.

Parents can claim disability benefit if the child is prescribed this drug.

So apart from affecting the mental health of the teenagers, this drug is causing heavy financial losses.

Comparative drugs like concerta, equasym are also not as safe as these were thought to be.

MODERN CONCEPTS ON BIRTH PILLS

Lot has been written on birth pills about its side effects in certain women, such as obesity, too much enlargement of breasts, high blood pressure, deep venous thrombosis, retinal changes.

Recent research paper in journal Trends in Ecology and Evolution, by Dr. Alexanrda Alvergne, from University of Sheffield shows that over a period of time birth pills affect the sexual inclination of women towards the opposite sex.

It is said women are more attracted to masculine men during fertile period and pills affect the fertile period by affecting the hormonal changes.

According to Dr. Alexandra, on days when women are not fertile, their tastes swing towards feminine, boyish faces.

According to her, the pill also changes their behaviour and alter women's view of male attractiveness.

Dr. Alvergne says the use of pill could influence women's ability to attract a mate by reducing her attractiveness to men.

Conclusively: Increasing number of studies suggest that the pill is likely to have an impact on human mating decisions and subsequent reproduction.

MODERN CONCEPTS ON SEX AND HEALTH

The recent concepts on health throw light, as to how important is the sex and timing of sex, as illustrated in the following researches.

British researchers at Queen University in Belfast have found, a good morning session, at least three times a week, decreases the risk of heart attack or stroke by half, and a regular session improves circulation, thereby reducing blood pressure.

According to New Scientist Journal's report, steamy session twice a week enhances IgA, an antibody that provides protection against microbes that multiply in body secretions. "The Sun" reports it burns 300 calories an hour that simultaneously diminishes the risk of developing diabetes.

The relation of sex and depression is demonstrated by the American studies, in 300 sexually active women whose partners did not use condoms, revealed they were less prone to depression. Sex increases the production of testosterone that provides stronger bones and muscles, thus helping to stave off osteoporosis.

A good morning session of sex can make the hair shine and skin glow by raising the output of oestrogens and other hormones which are associated with it.

According to Yale School of Medicine, researchers having morning sex can aid in averting endometrosis.

◆◆◆

19.

HOMEOPATHY AND STEROIDS

Many patients question use of steroids in Homeopathy. I am enclosing the reprint from renowned Homeopathy which gives the reply to those who question Homeopathy and steroid's use in it.

A lady asked a friend of mine if he could guide her to any good homeopath in the vicinity. He told her about me. 'Does your friend give powders?' asked the lady. 'Yes, occasionally,' answered my friend. 'Then I will never go to him, he must be giving steroids,' concluded the lady. Another lady who recently shifted to Delhi from Chandigarh was told by her homeopath back at Chandigarh to be wary of the homeopaths of Delhi as all of them used steroids according to the gentleman.

Rumours infest the public psyche today about the presence of steroids in homeopathic medicines. Had ignorance been bliss for these miserable beings, I would never have tried to bring them out of it, but I see so many people suffering and not trying homeopathy for things so easily curable that I could not help writing this article.

THE TRUTH ABOUT STEROIDS

'Steroids affect your heart. Steroids abuse has been associated with cardiovascular diseases, including heart attack and stroke. These heart problems can even happen to athletes under the age of 30.

Steroids affect your appearance in both sexes. Steroids can cause male pattern baldness, cysts, acne and oily hair and skin, jaundice (yellowness of skin), swelling of feet and ankles, aching joints, had breath nervousness and trembling. For girls, side effects can be growth of facial hair, deepened voice, breast size reduction. For boys, baldness, development of breasts, importance.

Steroids affect your mood, it can make you angry and hostile for no reason, there are recorded cases of murder attributed to intense anger from its use.

Side effects of oral steroids, taken daily, for long periods of time and/or in high dose, can be serious and may take a long time to go away once the medication is stopped. The most common side effect of steroids appears once the medication is stopped. The most common side effect of steroids taken for a short-time is an increased appetite. Some people also have more energy, feel a sense of well being, and have trouble sleeping, while others feel sad or irritable.

THE TRUTH ABOUT HOMEOPATHY

It is common knowledge that homeopathic medicines do not produce any such side effects. If any, the side effects in homepathy are only all positive. If you feel generally better after taking a homeopathic medicine that does not mean the medicine contains steroids. It happens because most of the polychrest medicines (a medicine of many uses) have a broad sphere of action and they affect almost every part of human body, including the endocrine system and an improved hormone balance and a generally improved health which gives the feeling of general well being. It is the first sign that the medicine is working well and is right for the patient; and ideally, this feeling should not be temporary like in case of artificial hormones.

TASTE OF STEROIDS

Masking the taste of steroids is not easy. Ever tasted the stuff yourself? It truly is vile. Oral steroids can be taken as pills or syrup. Steroid medicine has a bitter taste. Swallow the pills quickly and do not hold them in your mouth. The syrup also has a bitter taste or after taste and is best swallowed quickly. It is best not to take this medicine on an empty stomach. Interestingly, homeopathic medicines are anything but bitter and can be taken on an empty stomach; rather patients are encouraged to take the first dose in the morning on an empty stomach.

BUSTING THE MYTH

The powders used at times with homeopathic medicines have often been maligned as steroids. Nothing can be further from truth. The powder used in homeopathy is a benign substance derived from pure milk, usually imported from Holland, has a taste somewhat like glucose and is called sugar of milk. It is neutral in nature and has a long shelf life. The only purpose of the powder is to keep the medicine intact and save it from moisture etc. It also increases the efficacy of the dose as it sticks to the tongue and gives the body extra time to react to the medicine.

Some people say that the mother tinctures some homeopaths give contain steroids. First of all, I would like to mention that the use of mother tinctures internally is not recommended. Only one in ten thousand prescriptions by a true classical homeopath might need some occasional dose, if at all of any tincture.

One thing to be kept in mind is that we regularly get patients with ill-effects of steroids where we have to both detoxify the body and cure the patients. One cannot expect us to treat the side effects of steroids with steroids again. A lady who had gained about thirty-two kilos of weight after taking steroids, lost it within three-four months under our treatment and got relieved of the asthma as well, for which she was given steroids by doctors.

For us homeopaths, a case generally starts where conventional medicine fails to give a breakthrough. So any improvement a patient feels with homeopathic medicines remains a mystery for many. Medicine and teaching used to be missions, once we converted these into professions, profits and losses became part and parcel of these, like any other profession. The stupendous resurgence of homeopathy and its growing popularity across all strata of society is alarming for many. For people with vested interests, spreading rumours to sabotage homeopathy is only natural but before believing them, a patient should at least try to know the facts. Knowledge was never so freely available as today.

Homeopaths must understand that transparency can only add to their credibility, a patient has every right to know what he/she is given and why.

By Dr. Shikhar Kaushal (Founder Director, Panacea Homeopathic Clinic) and Dr. Shubhangee Kaushal (Former Registrar, NHMC, Delhi). For more information visit www.phc.in or Call 9810094369.

Panacea Homeopathic Clinic, L-22/7 Basement, Phase II, Dlf City, Near Private Hospital, Gurgaon-122002, India.

◆◆◆

20. DEBILITY

The debility (lassitude) or feeling physically or mentally tired. It could be both or only physical or only mental.

It is essential in homeopathy to analyse the exact cause unlike just giving vitamins for physical or brain tonics (like tranquillisers) for mental depression. As they do in allopathy.

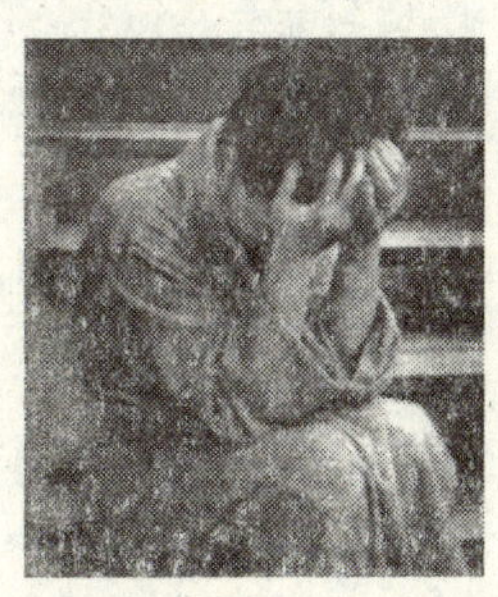

A few of the following cases treated with homeopathy after they had loads of vitamins did not work.

Allopathy

Any educated person realises that certain vitamins are harmful if taken in overdoses or for prolonged periods. Some vitamins are water soluble which if taken in excess are excreted. However fat soluble vitamins can be harmful if taken for too long period.

It is some of the minerals which if taken in doses exceeding the safe upper limit can be very harmful.

The word Antioxidant became very popular with public and pharmaceutics were exploiting.

I have seen cases of iron cirrhosis of liver and severe gastric problems with zinc and silicon, taken for long periods. They are damaging to the kidneys and liver, leaving-a-side gastritis and constipation for which these patients take antacids which cause calcium deficiency for which they take allopathic calcium which itself cause kidney stones if taken in high doses, or for prolonged periods.

Homeopathy

Very specific and individualised with physiological improvement in their well-being.

The following cases treated, are ample proof of beneficial effect of homeo-remedies:

1. Jet lag weakness or after strenuous excercise–arnica, bellis perenis and rhus tox are of unquestionable benefit.
2. Physical weakness after games in athletes-Arnica, ruta and rhus tox-because all the elements like muscle, ligaments are involved.
3. Physical debility in old age after excluding other causes, Curare and baryta carb are of immense benefit.
4. Physical debility after intercourse, selenium, acid phos and agnus are of unquestionable value.
5. Prostration, both physical and mental are best dealt with Picric acid and acid phos.
6. Debility during nursing or after diarrhoea, vomiting, there is no comparison to carbo veg 200 and china 200.

7. Debility due to loss of sleep as professional or factory workers on night shifts are best treated with cocculus.

8. Weakness following influenza with humming noises, there is no comparison to Nat. Salicylate.

9. Debility due to Prolapse uterus, leucorrhoea-Aletris F and Helonias can circumvent threes symptoms.

10. Mental strain weakness can be dealt with kaliphos rather than giving allopathic tranquillisers which will cause sedation.

11. Menopausal physical and mental weakness can be treated with ignatia, sepia and kali phos and if the woman is of violent temperament then Lachesis high potency will overcome.

12. Debility due to hot weather, there is no comparison to Natrum carb.

13. Mental and physical weakness in women due to sexual frustration or deprivation of sexual satisfaction, I have seen very good results with onosmodium and agnus.

◆◆◆

21.

WATER RETENTION VERSUS OBESITY

This is a bugbear for women. I have seen occurring much more frequently in women than men. Firstly, I want to make the women realise that what they attribute as obesity is more often water retention, rather than obesity, of course it gives appearance of obesity.

Secondly, the common cause of this water retention is allopathic drugs given for various ailment, the patient does not realise its long-term side effects.

Following facts about these drugs will make the women realise what they are heading to.

After they become obese or overweight due to water retention, they forget about the original illness and worry more about their overweight and go into depression.

To me they have come at a stage when they became tremendously obese, depression and irregular periods and loss of sleep.

Drugs which are commonly the culprit are as follows:

1. Most painkillers like brufen, voveran, diclofenac, advil, flexon, ibugesic.

2. Most of the harmone used to initiate the missed periods or birth pills.
3. Steroids are the most notorious for causing water retention leaving aside other side effects.

Allopathy

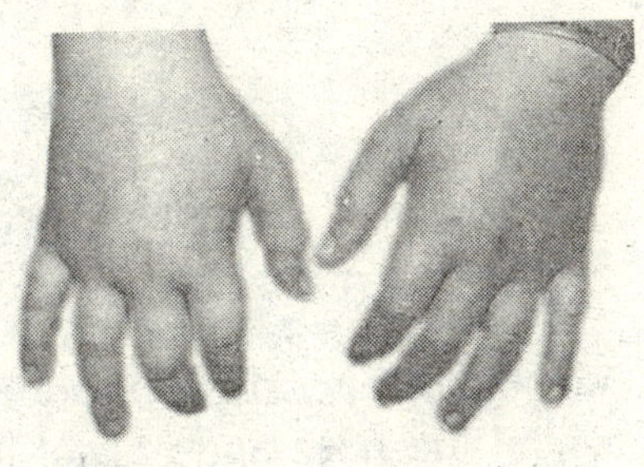

Treatment for Water Retention: Dytide or lasix are the common diuretics used. One should not forget about potassium depletion with lasix leading to extreme weakness and ecg changes in heart. To counteract potassium depletion, giving potassium by mouth leads to acidity. Continuing such treatment is bad for the kidney. Water loss leads to constipation and extreme dryness of mouth.

By these diuretics there is excretion of other minerals and salts leading to electrolyte imbalance.

Homeopathy

The combination of apis, apocyn and squilla are of unquestionable value. In severe cases I use Aegle follia and Marm. If the thyroid is affected by the hormonal treatment for amenorrhoea or heavy periods, then homeo. Thyroid preparation can be given. It is pity many women start dieting to reduce weight, while it is water retention than deposition of fat alone. Sometimes it is both then fat dissolving remedies can be given. Fat dissolving remedies in allopathy are fraught with dangerous side effects.

◆◆◆

22.

ADENOIDS AND DENTISTRY

Adenoid is also called nasopharyngeal tonsil. Its location is behind the nose and palate. It is present in every child and starts regressing after the age of 7 years.

Many people are under the impression that its presence is abnormal.

It is the size of adenoids which make it abnormal. The adenoids is a lymphoid tissue. It becomes enlarged due to infection, often associated with sinus infection or enlarges as a part of tonsil ring.

The enlarged tonsils often cause symptoms like snoring and mouth breathing and if it remains so then it affects the dental development which grow as deformed needing orthodental treatment.

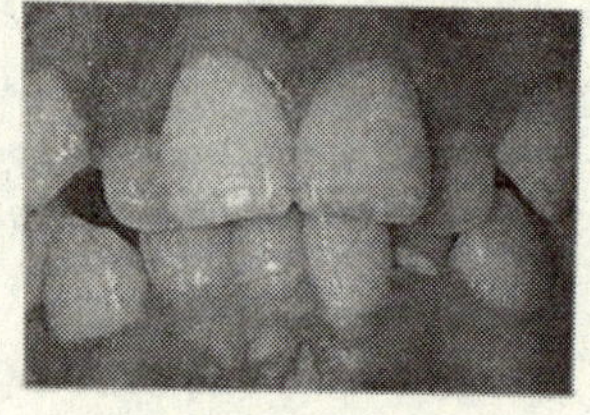

The orthodental treatment has become a fashion these days with elite class of public and dentists.

As an ENT surgeon, I would like to clarify some misunderstandings in public mind.

In India, parents are not willing to get operated for adenoids, if the child is even 4-6 years of age, despite the fact the hypertrophied adenoids are causing middle ear infection, mouth breathing, snoring and other complications.

For record, I would like to mention, the youngest I operated was six-month-old child in UK, because of middle ear deafness and infection.

If the parents wait till the age of 13 years or later, then irreversible damage and complication to ear, teeth and facial deformity is already done.

Allopathy

There are no medicines or antibiotics which are going to help. Depending upon the case, surgical removal gives miraculous results, provided if there is associated sinus infection that must be dealt with, which I feel most surgeons in India are reluctant to operate sinus in children.

However, small to medium size adenoids, I have cured with homeopathy with excellent results.

Homeopathy

Potency is selected with experience, I have been very happy the results I had with agraphis nutans and calcarea phos.

LOCK JAW

This condition, even the layman knows well but what they don't know or most of the doctors do not know the cause. In my experience the common causes of this condition are:

1. Rheumatic arthritis of the T.M. joints.
2. Keeping the mouth open for prolonged periods for dental

treatment leads to dysarthrosis of T.M. joint, leading subsequently to lock jaw.

3. Difficult intubation while giving general anaesthesia, especially patients suffering from C. spondylosis, leads to T.M. joint dysarthrosis thus leading to lock jaw.

Allopathy

I remember lot of these cases used to come in casualty in UK and I have to set the joint right under general anaesthesia.

One must not underestimate the fact that with advancing age it becomes difficult to set the joint owing to stiffness of spine.

Homeopathy

Magnesium phos and angustra and colocynth are excellent antispasmotics.

◆◆◆

23.

VARICOSE VEINS

This condition where there is loss of elasticity of leg veins leading to pooling of venous blood in the superficial veins of legs.

The appearance is of bluish and patient complains of heaviness of legs especially on standing.

This is common amongst women than men and common where the profession of women involves standing for long hours.

This must be distinguished from deep venous thrombosis (D.V.T) the chapter I have already dealt. The D.V.T is more serious in nature than V.V (varicose veins)

Allopathy

The common treatment in early cases is to inject sclerosing agents. In advance cases stripping is a very popular operation, but chances of recurrence even after operation are plenty.

Homeopathy

I have to deal many cases who had operation twice still the varicose veins have relapsed.

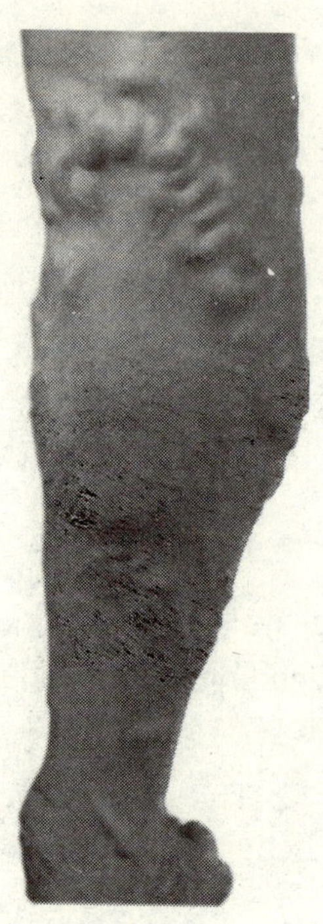

My common treatment in such cases is either singly or combination of the following remedies:

Hammamelis, aesculus, secale and pilsatilla.

Case: This is the worst case of a cook in someone's house who had very severe varicose veins with varicose ulcers, he had been operated twice, before he came to me.

On the basis of pathology I gave him calendula, arnica, lachesis and belladonna, he had a magical relief.

He had recurrence of it again after five years when he was working in a factory standing, three hundred miles away from Delhi, I gave him one dose of sulphur 1M followed by above combination. He has recovered fully at the time of writing his case.

◆◆◆

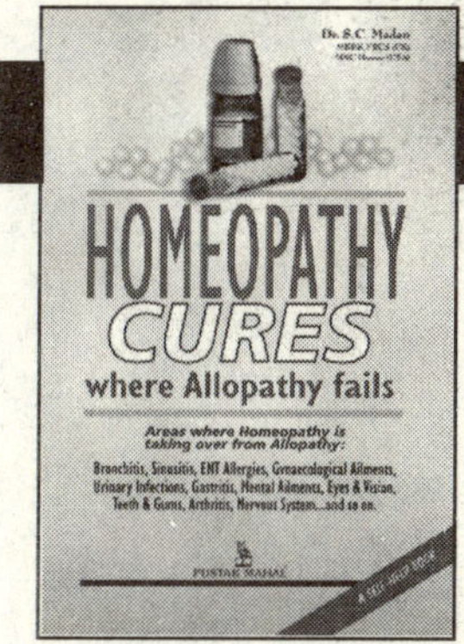

By the Same Author

HOMEOPATHY CURES

where Allopathy fails

– Dr. S. C. Madan

True, there's no substitute for Allopathy. With its life-saving drugs, antibiotics and surgery, it is the only answer to a range of critical illnesses and dreaded diseases. But despite extensive advancement and research in the field, Allopathy is unable to provide cure for a number of ailments. In this respect, Homeopathy has shown effective and proven results.

"Very often, the side effects caused due to the use of an allopathic drug are worse than the disease for which the drug had been administered," says the author, who is eminently qualified to compare the two sciences (Allopathy and Homeopathy). In this masterly, first of its kind book, the author lists specific ailments to prove his case. For instance, wherein chronic sinusitis, decongestants like Coldarin, Action 500, Actified, Cetrizine, etc., simply mask the symptoms without treating the cause, Kali Bio, Belladona, Kali Sulph and Calcarea Sulph provide effective cure. In cases of Skin Allergy, where dermatologists suggest anti-allergic treatment, Natrum Mur 1M can provide a permanent cure. Homeopathy can also be an effective treatment for Menorrhagia at menopause, which is otherwise treated with hormone replacement treatment, Gynae CVP, Dicyene and hysterectomy. Surgery can be avoided by Homeopathy in conditions like Prolapse uterus, Piles, Warts, Corns, etc.

In addition, the book lists specific Homeopathic medicines and treatment given in different cases- besides a section on frequently asked questions.